Understanding
Regression Analysis

Understanding Regression Analysis

Michael Patrick Allen

Washington State University
Pullman, Washington

Plenum Press • New York and London

Library of Congress Cataloging-in-Publication Data

Allen, Michael Patrick.
    Understanding regression analysis / Michael Patrick Allen.
        p.   cm.
    Includes bibliographical references and index.
    ISBN 0-306-45648-6
    1. Regression analysis.   I. Title.
QA278.2.A434   1997
519.5'36--dc21   97-20373
                                                           CIP

ISBN 0-306-45648-6

© 1997 Plenum Press, New York
A Division of Plenum Publishing Corporation
233 Spring Street, New York, N. Y. 10013

http://www.plenum.com

Printed in the United States of America

Preface

This book is intended to introduce readers who know relatively little about statistics and who have only a basic understanding of mathematics to one of the most powerful techniques in all of statistics: regression analysis. Regression analysis is one of the most widely used techniques in statistics because it can provide answers to many different analytical questions. Although regression analysis is used widely, it is not always used correctly. Unfortunately, many researchers use regression analysis without understanding either the basic logic or the statistical intricacies of this technique. It is hardly surprising, then, that regression analysis is often misused and its results misinterpreted.

This introduction to regression analysis requires only a rudimentary understanding of mathematics and statistics. Indeed, it requires only that the reader has some familiarity with basic algebra and some understanding of probability. This book proceeds on the assumption that it is possible to understand much of regression analysis without fully comprehending all of the mathematical proofs and statistical theory that underpin this technique. Although it assumes that the reader has only a basic background in mathematics, this book does attempt to introduce the reader to many of the fundamental conventions and operations of matrix algebra. A familiarity with matrix algebra not only renders regression analysis more comprehensible, it also enables the reader to understand more advanced multivariate statistical techniques.

The logic of this book is relatively straightforward. It reviews descriptive statistics using vector notation and presents the components of the simple regression model. Only then does it discuss the logic of sampling distributions and simple hypothesis testing. Next, it presents the basic operations of matrix algebra and develops the properties of the multiple regression model. It then goes on to examine the logic of testing compound hypotheses and the application of the regression model to the analysis of variance and analysis of covariance. Finally, it discusses a series of more advanced and specialized topics in regression analysis such as structural equation models and influence statistics.

This book seeks to provide the reader with an intuitive understanding of regression analysis. Consequently, it defers any discussion of issues of statistical inference until the reader has gained some grasp of the purely descriptive properties of the regression model. Indeed, many of the more complicated issues associated with statistical inference are discussed in only the most general terms. Mathematical derivations of some of the most important and most accessible properties of the regression model are presented in appendices. Moreover, this book does not include many of the equations typically found in discussions of regression analysis. One of the advantages of the regression model is that there are many mathematical relationships among the various quantities associated with this model. These mathematical properties may be useful to the trained statistician but they only serve to confuse the average reader. Finally, this book demonstrates the properties of the regression model using empirical examples that comprise only a few cases. As the reader will eventually discover, statistical analysis is not very useful in extremely small samples. However, examples comprising only a few cases enable the reader to follow more closely the calculations required to compute the various statistical measures.

Any competent statistician is likely to find this introduction to regression analysis overly simplistic. Indeed, many topics and issues that are near and dear to the hearts of statisticians, such as the power of statistical tests, have simply been ignored in this book. The omission of these issues from this presentation of regression analysis is not an attempt to belittle their importance. However, most of these issues are not especially relevant to the reader who wishes to gain no more than a basic understanding of regression analysis. Moreover, it is hoped that this book will provide the reader a firm understanding of the basic logic of regression analysis and that this understanding will provide them with the intellectual foundation to pursue more advanced issues and topics in statistics.

I am indebted to Scott Long, Tom Rotolo, Jean Stockard, and Lisa Barnett for their comments and suggestions on earlier drafts of this manuscript. They are not responsible, of course, for any remaining errors or omissions. Last but not least, I must acknowledge the contributions of many students whose responses to my lectures on regression analysis over the years gave shape to this book.

I wish to acknowledge that the empirical data used to demonstrate path analysis were taken from *Socioeconomic Background and Achievement* by Otis Duncan, David Featherman, and Beverly Duncan (New York: Seminar Press, 1972).

Contents

Understanding
Regression Analysis

CHAPTER 1

The Origins and Uses of Regression Analysis

Statistical techniques are tools that enable us to answer questions about possible patterns in empirical data. It is not surprising, then, to learn that many important techniques of statistical analysis were developed by scientists who were interested in answering very specific empirical questions. So it was with regression analysis. The history of this particular statistical technique can be traced back to late nineteenth-century England and the pursuits of a gentleman scientist, Francis Galton. Galton was born into a wealthy family that produced more than its share of geniuses; he and Charles Darwin, the famous biologist, were first cousins. During his lifetime, Galton studied everything from fingerprint classification to meteorology, but he gained widespread recognition primarily for his work on inheritance. His most important insight came to him while he was studying the inheritance of one of the most obvious of all human characteristics: height. In order to understand how the characteristic of height was passed from one generation to the next, Galton collected data on the heights of individuals and the heights of their parents. After constructing frequency tables that classified these individuals both by their height and by the average height of their parents, Galton came to the unremarkable conclusion that tall people usually had tall parents and short people usually had short parents. In other words, he found that one could predict, with some accuracy, the heights of individuals from the heights of their parents. The data on which he based his conclusions are presented, in a highly condensed form, in Table 1.1.

Table 1.1. Frequency Distribution of Heights of Adult Children by Average Heights of Parents

Average height of parents (in inches)	Height of adult child (in inches)				
	≤ 65	66-67	68-69	70-71	≥ 72
≥ 72	1	7	11	17	30
70-71	24	48	83	66	3
68-69	72	130	148	69	11
66-67	35	56	41	11	1
≤ 65	19	14	4	0	0

Source: Based on data published by Galton in 1886.

However, after studying these data in greater detail, Galton came to another, more remarkable, conclusion. Individuals who had tall parents were often taller than average, but they were usually not as tall as their parents. Conversely, individuals who had short parents were often shorter than average, but they too were usually not as short as their parents. Galton termed this pattern of inheritance "regression to the mean." By that, he meant that parents who were far from average on any characteristic, such as height, often had children who were closer to the average on that characteristic. In proposing his principle of the regression to the mean, Galton had not only discovered an important principle of genetics, he had also identified, quite inadvertently, two concepts that would become very important to the burgeoning field of statistics. The first concept had to do with developing a method for predicting the values of one quantitative variable, such as the heights of individuals, using the values of another quantitative variable, such as the heights of their parents. For example, even though there was some regression to the mean, the heights of individuals were related, in a general way, to the heights of their parents. Galton realized that it should be possible to develop a mathematical function to describe such a relationship between two quantitative variables. The second concept had to do with developing a method for assessing the lawfulness or regularity of any such relationship. Galton realized that some relationships might be more predictable than others. For example, the heights of individuals could not be predicted precisely from the heights of their parents. Galton referred to the degree of predictability in a relationship as the "closeness of co-relation." Regression and correlation were destined to become two of the most important concepts in statistics. Although he discovered these concepts, Galton was not able to provide exact mathematical definitions for either of them. The task of developing the precise mathematical formulas for regression and correlation was completed over the next few years by three English statisticians: Francis Edgeworth, Karl Pearson, and George Yule. They, in turn, relied heavily on mathematical proofs developed almost a century earlier by Carl Friedrich Gauss, who was interested in the problem of reconciling variations in astronomical observations.

Simple regression and correlation form the basis of what is generally referred to today as regression analysis. In general, regression analysis is a statistical technique that attempts to predict the values of one variable using the values of one or more other variables. By convention, the variable that we are trying to predict is called the dependent variable and the variables that we are using as predictors of that variable are called independent variables. For example, we might wish to explain the relationship between education, measured in years of formal schooling, and income. In this case, we would typically assume that income is the dependent variable and that education is the independent variable. For a number of reasons, there is a positive relationship between these two variables. Individuals who have more education than average usually have incomes that are above average. Conversely, individuals who have less education than average typically have incomes that are below average. Regression analysis allows us to estimate the form of this relationship between these two variables. In particular, it enables us to predict the level of income associated with each level of education. Regression analysis also allows us to assess how accurately an independent variable predicts a dependent variable. Specifically, it enables us to determine the proportion of the variation in the dependent variable that can be accounted for by the variation in the independent variable. For example, we cannot predict the incomes of individuals exactly using their educations. Regression analysis allows us to examine simultaneously both the form of a relationship and the accuracy of a relationship. Last but not least, regression analysis can also tell us whether or not a particular relationship is statistically significant. In other words, it can tell us the probability that the relationship that we observe between two variables in a given sample also obtains in the population as a whole.

If these were the only questions that could be answered using regression analysis, it would hardly qualify as one of the most useful and powerful of all statistical techniques. Fortunately, it can do a great deal more. The real utility of regression analysis becomes apparent when we seek to examine relationships that involve more than one independent variable. This technique, known as multiple regression analysis, allows us to estimate the form and accuracy of a relationship between a dependent variable and several independent variables at once. In so doing, we can examine the effect of one independent variable on the dependent variable controlling for the effects of other independent variables. For example, using multiple regression analysis, we can examine the relationship between income and both education and gender. Specifically, we can estimate the form of the relationship between income and education, controlling for gender, and the form of the relationship between income and gender, controlling for income. Indeed, the main advantage of regression analysis is that it allows us to disentangle the relative effects on a dependent variable of two or more independent variables. We can also determine the accuracy of this relationship with two independent variables and compare it to the accuracy of the relationship with one independent variable. It is worth noting, in this regard, that multiple regression analysis also allows us to use independent variables, like gender, that are categorical rather than continuous variables. Consequently, multiple regression analysis can perform tasks associated with other statistical techniques, such as analysis of variance and analysis of covariance, that employ categorical independent variables.

Finally, it is important to bear in mind that regression analysis is nothing more than a mathematical model for describing and analyzing particular types of patterns in empirical data. Although regression analysis is arguably the most flexible and powerful analytical tool ever developed by statisticians, it has its limitations. In order to use regression analysis, we are forced to impose a specific set of assumptions on our data. Although these assumptions are not especially stringent, they are not necessarily appropriate for all problems. As a result, statisticians have developed a series of more advanced techniques for analyzing data that are not suited to ordinary regression analysis. For example, regression analysis requires a continuous dependent variable. As a result, statisticians have developed a series of more advanced techniques for analyzing data that are not suited to ordinary multiple regression analysis. In many cases, these advanced techniques, such as logistic regression, are merely extensions of the regression analysis model. Consequently, despite their mathematical complexities, these techniques can usually be understood by anyone who understands regression analysis. In any event, we must always be aware of the fact that statistical models, such as the regression model, never "emerge" from data. Instead, we simply "impose" these models and all of their attendant assumptions on our data. As the term suggests, a model is only a representation designed to display the basic structure of a more complex set of phenomena. In the end, we must be prepared to justify, on both theoretical and empirical grounds, our choice of a particular model to represent our data.

CHAPTER 2

Basic Matrix Algebra: Manipulating Vectors

Statistics is, of course, a branch of applied mathematics. Consequently, anyone who wishes to understand statistics must first understand basic mathematics. In the case of simple regression analysis, we only need to be familiar with ordinary algebra. However, if we wish to understand multiple regression analysis, we must be familiar with the basic conventions and operations of matrix algebra. Statisticians routinely employ matrix algebra to describe multivariate models such as multiple regression analysis because it enables them to manipulate large systems of equations using compact algebraic expressions. *Matrices consist of arrays of numbers or elements arranged in rows and columns.* We can begin to understand matrix algebra by learning to manipulate the simplest matrices of all: vectors. *A vector is an array consisting of a single row or column of numbers or elements.*

In regression analysis, we typically represent the observations on a single variable by a column vector. A column vector can be thought of as a matrix with N rows and one column (i.e., $N \times 1$). For example, four observations on a variable, x, can be represented by a single column vector, $\mathbf{x}$, as follows:

$$\mathbf{x} = \begin{bmatrix} x_1 \\ x_2 \\ x_3 \\ x_4 \end{bmatrix} = \begin{bmatrix} 2 \\ 4 \\ 6 \\ 8 \end{bmatrix}$$

In order to distinguish them from other algebraic quantities, we shall denote vectors with bold lower-case letters and matrices with bold upper-case letters.

One of the basic operations of matrix algebra is *transposition*. The transposition operation is represented by a single prime mark following the letter of the vector being transposed. In transposing a column vector into a row vector, each element of the column vector becomes the corresponding element of the row vector as follows:

$$\mathbf{x}' = \begin{bmatrix} x_1 & x_2 & x_3 & x_4 \end{bmatrix} = \begin{bmatrix} 2 & 4 & 6 & 8 \end{bmatrix}$$

A row vector can be thought of as a matrix with one row and N columns (i.e., 1 x N). Of course, it is possible to transpose a row vector into a column vector as follows:

$$(\mathbf{x}')' = \mathbf{x}$$

In this case, each element of the row vector becomes the corresponding element of the column vector.

In regression analysis, we must often add and subtract vectors of numbers. It is possible to add or subtract any two vectors as long as they are *conformable*. *Two vectors are conformable for addition or subtraction whenever they have the same dimensions.* For example, it is possible to add two column vectors whenever they have the same number of elements (i.e., N x 1 and N x 1). Conversely, it is possible to add two row vectors whenever they have the same number of elements (i.e., 1 x N and 1x N). However, it is not possible to add a column vector and a row vector, even if they have the same number of elements, because they have different dimensions (i.e., N x 1 and 1 x N)

In vector addition, the elements of the first vector are simply added to the corresponding elements of the second vector. For example, given the following column vectors:

$$\mathbf{x} = \begin{bmatrix} x_1 \\ x_2 \\ x_3 \\ x_4 \end{bmatrix} = \begin{bmatrix} 2 \\ 4 \\ 6 \\ 8 \end{bmatrix} \quad \text{and} \quad \mathbf{y} = \begin{bmatrix} y_1 \\ y_2 \\ y_3 \\ y_4 \end{bmatrix} = \begin{bmatrix} 2 \\ 0 \\ 2 \\ 0 \end{bmatrix}$$

the result of the addition of **x** and **y** is given by:

$$\mathbf{x} + \mathbf{y} = \begin{bmatrix} x_1 + y_1 \\ x_2 + y_2 \\ x_3 + y_3 \\ x_4 + y_4 \end{bmatrix} = \begin{bmatrix} 2 + 2 \\ 4 + 0 \\ 6 + 2 \\ 8 + 0 \end{bmatrix} = \begin{bmatrix} 4 \\ 4 \\ 8 \\ 8 \end{bmatrix}$$

We can, of course, add any number of vectors as long as they all have the same dimensions.

Similarly, in vector subtraction, the elements in the second vector are subtracted from the corresponding elements in the first vector. For example, given the same two vectors, the result of the subtraction of $\mathbf{y}$ from $\mathbf{x}$ is given by:

$$\mathbf{x} - \mathbf{y} = \begin{bmatrix} x_1 - y_1 \\ x_2 - y_2 \\ x_3 - y_3 \\ x_4 - y_4 \end{bmatrix} = \begin{bmatrix} 2 - 2 \\ 4 - 0 \\ 6 - 2 \\ 8 - 0 \end{bmatrix} = \begin{bmatrix} 0 \\ 4 \\ 4 \\ 8 \end{bmatrix}$$

It is worth noting that the addition or subtraction of row vectors is performed in precisely the same manner such that

$$\mathbf{x}' - \mathbf{y}' = \begin{bmatrix} x_1 - y_1 & x_2 - y_2 & x_3 - y_3 & x_4 - y_4 \end{bmatrix}$$

$$= \begin{bmatrix} 2 - 2 & 4 - 0 & 6 - 2 & 8 - 0 \end{bmatrix}$$

$$= \begin{bmatrix} 0 & 4 & 4 & 8 \end{bmatrix}$$

We could, of course, have obtained the same result by subtracting the two column vectors and transposing the result such that:

$$\mathbf{x}' - \mathbf{y}' = (\mathbf{x} - \mathbf{y})'$$

In regression analysis, we must often also multiply vectors of numbers by a single quantity. In matrix algebra, such a single quantity is known as a *scalar* or constant. Moreover, in matrix algebra, we distinguish between premultiplication and postmultiplication because the order in which scalars and vectors are multiplied is important. For example, it is permissible to premultiply a row vector by a scalar as follows:

$$a \, y' = \begin{bmatrix} ay_1 & ay_2 & ay_3 & ay_4 \end{bmatrix} = 2 \begin{bmatrix} 2 & 0 & 2 & 0 \end{bmatrix}$$

$$= \begin{bmatrix} (2)(2) & (2)(0) & (2)(2) & (2)(0) \end{bmatrix}$$

$$= \begin{bmatrix} 4 & 0 & 4 & 0 \end{bmatrix}$$

In short, each element of the row vector is multiplied by the scalar. This operation is permissible in matrix algebra because a scalar can be considered a matrix with one row and one column (i.e., 1 x 1) and a row vector can be considered a matrix with one row and several columns (i.e., 1 x N). Two matrices are conformable for multiplication if the number of columns in the premultiplying matrix is equal to the number of rows in the postmultiplying matrix. For the same reason, it is permissible to postmultiply a column vector by a scalar as follows:

$$y \, a = \begin{bmatrix} y_1 a \\ y_2 a \\ y_3 a \\ y_4 a \end{bmatrix} = \begin{bmatrix} 2 \\ 0 \\ 2 \\ 0 \end{bmatrix} 2 = \begin{bmatrix} (2)(2) \\ (0)(2) \\ (2)(2) \\ (0)(2) \end{bmatrix} = \begin{bmatrix} 4 \\ 0 \\ 4 \\ 0 \end{bmatrix}$$

However, it is not permissible in matrix algebra to either premultiply a column vector by a scalar or postmultiply a row vector by a scalar because the number of columns in the premultiplying matrix is not equal to the number of rows in the postmultiplying matrix. We can also divide a vector by a scalar by simply multiplying that vector by the inverse of that scalar as follows:

$$\frac{1}{a} \, y' = \begin{bmatrix} \frac{1}{a} y_1 & \frac{1}{a} y_2 & \frac{1}{a} y_3 & \frac{1}{a} y_4 \end{bmatrix}$$

$$= \frac{1}{2} \, y' = \frac{1}{2} \begin{bmatrix} 2 & 0 & 2 & 0 \end{bmatrix}$$

$$= \begin{bmatrix} \left(\frac{1}{2}\right)(2) & \left(\frac{1}{2}\right)(0) & \left(\frac{1}{2}\right)(2) & \left(\frac{1}{2}\right)(0) \end{bmatrix}$$

$$= \begin{bmatrix} 1 & 0 & 1 & 0 \end{bmatrix}$$

In addition, regression analysis often requires us to calculate the sum of the products of the elements in one vector and the corresponding elements in another vector. Two vectors are conformable for multiplication whenever the number of columns in the first vector is equal to the number of rows in the second vector. Therefore, we can premultiply a column vector by a row vector, or postmultiply a row vector by a column vector, whenever they have the same number of elements. This operation, which is known as the *scalar product* of two vectors, yields a scalar that is equal to the sum of the products of the elements in the corresponding vectors. For example, the scalar product $\mathbf{x'y}$ is computed as follows:

$$\mathbf{x'y} = x_1 y_1 + x_2 y_2 + x_3 y_3 + x_4 y_4 = \sum x_i y_i$$

$$= (2)(2) + (4)(0) + (6)(2) + (8)(0)$$

$$= 4 + 0 + 12 + 0 = 16$$

This quantity is sometimes referred to as the sum of the cross products of two variables. It is worth noting that the scalar product of two conformable vectors is not affected by the order of the vectors such that:

$$\mathbf{y'x} = y_1 x_1 + y_2 x_2 + y_3 x_3 + y_4 x_4 = \mathbf{x'y}$$

One special case of this operation involves premultiplying a column vector by its transpose. This operation, known as the *inner product* of a vector, yields a scalar that is equal to the sum of the squared elements in the vector. For example, the inner product $\mathbf{y'y}$ can be computed as follows:

$$\mathbf{y'y} = y_1^2 + y_2^2 + y_3^2 + y_4^2 = \sum y_i^2$$

$$= (2)(2) + (0)(0) + (2)(2) + (0)(0)$$

$$= 4 + 0 + 4 + 0 = 8$$

As we shall soon discover, these two quantities, the sum of the cross products of two variables and the sum of the squared values of a variable, are very important in regression analysis.

CHAPTER 3

The Mean and Variance
of a Variable

Much of regression analysis, indeed much of statistical analysis in general, involves the related concepts of mean and variance. The mean and the variance are known as "descriptive" statistics. They are summary measures that describe the basic characteristics of a distribution of numbers. The mean is a measure of central tendency. As such, it conveys information about the "center" or "midpoint" of a distribution of numbers. The variance is a measure of dispersion. It conveys information about the "spread" or "variability" of the numbers in a distribution around the mean. Together, the mean and the variance tell us a great deal about the distribution of any variable.

The mean is defined as the average of the observed values on a variable. Consequently, it is calculated by simply summing all of the observed values on a variable and dividing by the number of observations. Unfortunately, there is no simple operation in matrix algebra for summing all of the elements in a vector. However, we can achieve this result by obtaining the scalar product of a vector of numbers with a unit vector, whose elements are ones. Therefore, the mean of a variable, $\bar{x}$, can be expressed in matrix algebra as follows:

$$\text{Mean}(x) = \frac{1}{N}(\mathbf{u}'\mathbf{x}) = \frac{1}{N}\sum(1)(x_i)$$

$$= \frac{1}{N}\sum x_i = \bar{x}$$

where $\mathbf{u}'$ is the unit row vector of ones and $\mathbf{x}$ is the column vector of observations on variable x such that:

$$\mathbf{u}' = \begin{bmatrix} 1 & 1 & 1 & \cdots & 1 \end{bmatrix} \quad \text{and} \quad \mathbf{x} = \begin{bmatrix} x_1 \\ x_2 \\ x_3 \\ \vdots \\ x_n \end{bmatrix}$$

The variance is defined as the average of all the squared deviations of the observed values from the mean of a variable. As such, it is calculated by simply summing all of the squared deviations from the mean. In matrix algebra notation, the sum of the squared deviations from the mean for a variable, known simply as its *sum of squares*, can be expressed as follows:

$$SS(x) = (\mathbf{x} - \bar{\mathbf{x}})'(\mathbf{x} - \bar{\mathbf{x}}) = \sum (x_i - \bar{x})$$

where

$$\mathbf{x} - \bar{\mathbf{x}} = \begin{bmatrix} x_1 \\ x_2 \\ x_3 \\ \vdots \\ x_n \end{bmatrix} - \begin{bmatrix} \bar{x} \\ \bar{x} \\ \bar{x} \\ \vdots \\ \bar{x} \end{bmatrix} = \begin{bmatrix} x_1 - \bar{x} \\ x_2 - \bar{x} \\ x_3 - \bar{x} \\ \vdots \\ x_n - \bar{x} \end{bmatrix}$$

Consequently, the variance of a variable, s^2, can be obtained by dividing its sum of squares by the number of observations as follows:

$$Var(x) = \frac{1}{N} SS(x) = \frac{1}{N} (\mathbf{x} - \bar{\mathbf{x}})'(\mathbf{x} - \bar{\mathbf{x}})$$

$$= \frac{1}{N} \sum (x_i - \bar{x})^2 = s^2$$

As these equations suggest, it can be a very laborious task to compute the deviations from the mean for a variable. Fortunately, we can derive a more convenient computational equation for the variance of a variable using matrix algebra. To begin with, we can decompose the sum of squares by performing the indicated vector multiplication operations as follows:

$$SS(x) = (x - \bar{x})'(x - \bar{x}) = x'(x - \bar{x}) - \bar{x}'(x - \bar{x})$$

$$= x'x - x'\bar{x} - \bar{x}'x + \bar{x}'\bar{x}$$

$$= \sum x_i^2 - \sum x_i \bar{x} - \sum \bar{x} x_i + \sum \bar{x}^2$$

This equation can be greatly simplified by noting that the last three quantities are all equal to one another as follows:

$$\sum x_i \bar{x} = \sum \bar{x} x_i = \bar{x} \sum x_i$$

$$= \bar{x}(N\bar{x}) = N\bar{x}^2$$

$$\sum \bar{x}^2 = N\bar{x}^2$$

In short, these quantities are equal to the number of cases times the square of the mean. Therefore, the sum of squares can be reduced to the sum of the squared observed values minus a quantity equal to the number of cases times the squared mean such that:

$$SS(x) = \sum x_i^2 - N\bar{x}^2 = x'x - \bar{x}'\bar{x}$$

This implies that the variance of a variable is equal to the average of the squared observed values minus the squared mean of these values such that:

$$Var(x) = \frac{1}{N} SS(x) = \frac{1}{N}(x'x - \bar{x}'\bar{x})$$

$$= \frac{1}{N}\sum(x_i^2 - N\bar{x}^2) = \frac{1}{N}\sum x_i^2 - \bar{x}^2$$

We can demonstrate the computations for obtaining the mean and variance using a simple example with four observations on variable x such that:

$$\mathbf{x} = \begin{bmatrix} 6 \\ 8 \\ 10 \\ 16 \end{bmatrix}$$

Therefore, the mean of variable x is computed as follows:

$$\bar{x} = \frac{1}{N}(\mathbf{u}'\mathbf{x}) = \frac{1}{N}\sum x_i$$

$$= \frac{1}{4}(6 + 8 + 10 + 16) = \frac{1}{4}(40) = 10$$

If we wish to compute the variance of variable x, we can do so in one of two ways. The first is to compute the deviations of variable x from its mean as follows:

$$\mathbf{x} - \bar{\mathbf{x}} = \begin{bmatrix} 6 \\ 8 \\ 10 \\ 16 \end{bmatrix} - \begin{bmatrix} 10 \\ 10 \\ 10 \\ 10 \end{bmatrix} = \begin{bmatrix} -4 \\ -2 \\ 0 \\ 6 \end{bmatrix}$$

In short, we obtain the mean deviations by subtracting the mean from each observed value. Next, we obtain the average squared value of these deviations from the mean as follows:

$$\text{Var}(x) = \frac{1}{N}(\mathbf{x} - \bar{\mathbf{x}})'(\mathbf{x} - \bar{\mathbf{x}}) = \frac{1}{N}\sum(x_i - \bar{x})^2$$

$$= \frac{1}{4}\left[(-4)^2 + (-2)^2 + (0)^2 + (6)^2\right]$$

$$= \frac{1}{4}(16 + 4 + 0 + 36) = \frac{1}{4}(56) = 14$$

An alternative way of obtaining the same result is to employ the computational equation for the variance of a variable such that:

$$= \frac{1}{4} \left[(6)^2 + (8)^2 + (10)^2 + (16)^2 \right] - (10)^2$$

$$= \frac{1}{4} (36 + 64 + 100 + 256) - 100$$

$$= \frac{1}{4} (456) - 100 = 114 - 100 = 14$$

Consequently, we can compute the variance of a variable without actually computing the deviations of each observation from the mean.

One of the most important properties of the mean, as a measure of central tendency, is that the sum of all the deviations from the mean is equal to zero. This can be seen clearly in our example such that:

$$\Sigma(x_i - \bar{x}) = \mathbf{u}'(\mathbf{x} - \bar{\mathbf{x}})$$

$$= (1)(-4) + (1)(-2) + (1)(0) + (1)(6)$$

$$= (-4) + (-2) + (0) + (6) = 0$$

It is in this sense, then, that the mean is often interpreted as the "center of gravity" of a distribution. The sum of all the deviations above the mean is equal to the sum of all the deviations below the mean.

Finally, it must be pointed out that these equations for the mean and the variance of a variable are used to compute the value of these statistics in a sample. Moreover, the sample mean of a variable yields an unbiased estimate of the mean of that variable in the population. A sample estimate of a population parameter is said to be "unbiased" if the average value of that estimate, over a large number of samples, is equal to the population parameter. However, the sample variance of a variable yields a biased estimate of the variance of that variable the population. Specifically, the sample variance systematically underestimates the population variance, especially in small samples. Fortunately, we can obtain an unbiased estimate of the population variance of a variable by dividing the sample sum of squares by the quantity $N - 1$ instead of N, where N is the size of the sample.

CHAPTER 4

Regression Models and Linear Functions

Regression analysis proceeds from one basic assumption. Specifically, this technique assumes, at least initially, that the relationships between the variables in the analysis are "linear." For example, simple regression analysis assumes that one variable can be expressed, at least approximately, as a linear function of another variable. A linear function is simply one of many possible mathematical functions that one might employ to predict one variable using another variable, and it is not immediately apparent why we should favor a linear function over other functions. Perhaps the best reason for describing the relationship between two variables in terms of a linear function is its simplicity. Linear functions are less complex than most other mathematical functions, and the principle of parsimony in science suggests that, other things being equal, we should choose simple explanations over more complex ones. Linear functions are also often most appropriate because many theoretical statements in the social sciences can be readily translated into the form of a linear function. For example, stratification theory suggests that income increases directly with increases in education. This theoretical statement can easily be translated into the more formal proposition that income is a linear function of education. Of course, the most important consideration is simply how well a linear function fits the empirical data on education and income.

In order to understand the nature of linear functions and linear relationships between variables, it is best to start with a simple example. The simplest linear function is one involving only two variables, a dependent variable and an independent variable. As the terminology suggests, the value of the dependent variable depends on the value of the independent variable. Conversely, the value of the independent variable is independent of the value of the dependent variable. In short, the independent variable is the cause and the dependent variable is the effect. From a purely mathematical perspective, regression analysis assumes that the values of the dependent variable can be expressed, at least approximately, as a linear function of the values of the independent variable. *A linear relationship is one in which the change in the dependent variable produced by a given change in the independent variable is constant.* Whenever the rate of change between two variables is not constant, the relationship between them is nonlinear.

Let us consider a hypothetical example of the relationship between education and income for four individuals. We can represent the data on these two variables for these four individuals using two vectors, each containing four elements. In regression analysis, we typically denote the dependent variable by the letter y and the independent variable by the letter x. Therefore, the vector **y** contains the observed values for these four individuals on the dependent variable, income, expressed in thousands of dollars per year, such that:

$$\mathbf{y} = \begin{bmatrix} y_1 \\ y_2 \\ y_3 \\ y_4 \end{bmatrix} = \begin{bmatrix} 16 \\ 22 \\ 29 \\ 35 \end{bmatrix}$$

Conversely, the vector **x** contains the corresponding observed values on the independent variable, education, expressed in years of schooling, such that:

$$\mathbf{x} = \begin{bmatrix} x_1 \\ x_2 \\ x_3 \\ x_4 \end{bmatrix} = \begin{bmatrix} 12 \\ 16 \\ 14 \\ 18 \end{bmatrix}$$

In order to examine this relationship, we can begin by plotting the location of each of these four individuals in a two-dimensional space. By convention, we plot the values of y along the vertical axis and the values of x along the horizontal axis. The coordinates of each point are given

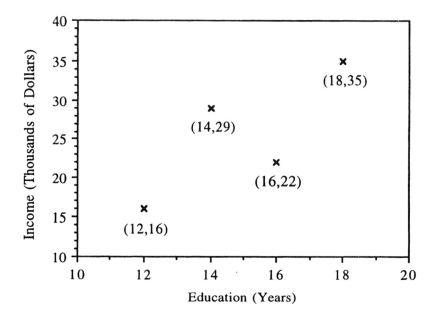

Figure 4.1. Plot of Income and Education

with the x value first and the y value second. A plot of these four obser-vations in such a two-dimensional space is presented in Figure 4.1. For example, the first observation is represented by the point that corresponds to 12 on the x axis and 16 on the y axis. A visual inspection of these four data points indicates that they fall roughly in a line such that income increases with education. The goal of regression analysis is to determine the parameters of the linear function that best describes the joint distribution of these two variables.

A simple linear function contains two parameters. The first is the slope coefficient, represented by b, and the second is the intercept, repre-sented by a. Consequently, the linear function for the predicted value of y in terms of the observed value of x is given by the following equation:

$$\hat{y}_i \ = \ a \ + \ bx_i$$

This same equation can be represented in matrix algebra as follows:

$$\hat{\mathbf{y}} = \mathbf{u}a + \mathbf{x}b$$

Note that there is a "hat" over the y to indicate that the linear function only gives us the "predicted" values of y. In almost every instance using empirical data, there will be some disparity between these predicted values of y and the corresponding observed values of y.

One of the most important things we want to know about this linear function is the value of the slope coefficient, b, which measures how much income can be expected to increase as a result of a one unit increase in education. The slope coefficient of a linear function measures the rate of change in y associated with a given change in x such that:

$$b \approx \frac{\Delta y}{\Delta x} \approx \frac{y_j - y_i}{x_j - x_i}$$

In the absence of any statistical criterion for choosing one value of the slope coefficient over another, we might choose an appropriate value simply from a visual inspection of the graph. It turns out that we can plot a regression line that is equidistant from all of the observations if we set the slope coefficient as follows:

$$b = 1.5$$

In other words, income can be expected to increase by $1,500 with every one year increase in education.

It is important to note that the intercept is determined by the slope coefficient. If we want our linear function to pass through the point representing the means on both variables, we must set the intercept to be equal to the difference between the mean of the observed y values and the product of the slope coefficient and the mean of the observed x values as follows:

$$a = \bar{y} - b\bar{x} = 25.5 - (1.5)(15)$$

$$= 25.5 - 22.5 = 3.0$$

This equation for the intercept may seem somewhat arbitrary but it is not. It is entirely logical that a regression line should pass through the centers of the distributions of both the dependent and the independent variables.

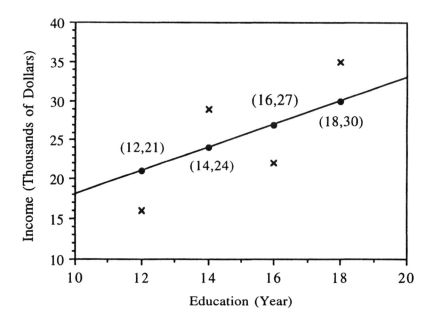

Figure 4.2. Plot of Arbitrary Regression Function

Given the slope coefficient of 1.5 and the intercept of 3.0, we can compute the predicted y values associated with the observed x values as follows:

$$\hat{\mathbf{y}} = \mathbf{u}a + \mathbf{x}b$$

$$= \begin{bmatrix} 1 \\ 1 \\ 1 \\ 1 \end{bmatrix} 3.0 + \begin{bmatrix} 12 \\ 16 \\ 14 \\ 18 \end{bmatrix} 1.5 = \begin{bmatrix} 3 \\ 3 \\ 3 \\ 3 \end{bmatrix} + \begin{bmatrix} 18 \\ 24 \\ 21 \\ 27 \end{bmatrix} = \begin{bmatrix} 21 \\ 27 \\ 24 \\ 30 \end{bmatrix}$$

The graph of the line corresponding to this linear function can be plotted as shown in Figure 4.2. It should be apparent that all of the predicted values of y fall precisely on the line representing the linear function. Of course, the observed values of y fall somewhat above and below these predicted values.

CHAPTER 5

Errors of Prediction and
Least-Squares Estimation

From a statistical point of view, the goal of simple regression analysis is to find the slope coefficient and the intercept for the linear function that best describes the relationship between two variables. The slope coefficient, which is also known as the regression coefficient, is important because it measures the amount of change in the dependent variable associated with a one unit change in the independent variable. In the example used earlier, a regression coefficient of 1.5 suggests that income can be expected to increase by $1,500 for every one year increase in education. However, this arbitrary regression coefficient is only one of any number of regression coefficients that one might employ to describe these data. The best way to choose between alternative regression coefficients is to compare the errors of prediction associated with different linear regression equations. *Errors of prediction are defined as the differences between the observed values of the dependent variable and the predicted values for that variable obtained using a given regression equation and the observed values of the independent variable.*

In order to compare the results obtained from different regression coefficients, we begin by calculating the errors of prediction associated with our arbitrary regression coefficient as follows:

$$\mathbf{e} = \mathbf{y} - \mathbf{\hat{y}} = \begin{bmatrix} 16 \\ 22 \\ 29 \\ 35 \end{bmatrix} - \begin{bmatrix} 21 \\ 27 \\ 24 \\ 30 \end{bmatrix} = \begin{bmatrix} -5 \\ -5 \\ 5 \\ 5 \end{bmatrix}$$

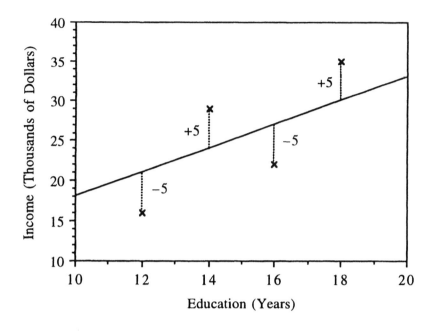

Figure 5.1. Errors of Arbitrary Regression Function

Obviously, the regression equation based on this arbitrary regression coefficient provides only very approximate predictions of the observed y values. However, it has the virtue of being equally inaccurate for all observations.

It is worth noting that each error of prediction can be plotted graphically as the perpendicular distance between each observed value and its predicted value along the regression line. For example, using the regression equation with a regression coefficient of 1.5 and an intercept of 3.0, the first individual, who has 12 years of education, has a predicted income of $21,000. However, the observed income of that individual is $16,000. In other words, that individual earns $5,000 less than we predicted using this regression equation. This error of prediction is shown in Figure 5.1 as the distance between the observed value and the predicted value on the regression line. The errors of prediction for the remaining three observations can be plotted in the same manner.

It might seem, at first glance, that the best way of comparing how well different regression equations fit a given set of data would be to compare the sum of the errors associated with each regression equation.

However, this simple procedure is not satisfactory because the errors of prediction for any regression equation sum to zero. This property obtains by virtue of the manner in which we calculated the value of the intercept. Alternatively, we might measure the adequacy of a regression equation by computing the sum of the absolute values of the errors of prediction associated with that equation. However, such a procedure is somewhat arbitrary. Conversely, we might measure the adequacy of a regression equation by computing the sum of the squared errors of prediction associated with that equation. This criterion is not entirely arbitrary because it is similar to the procedure that we use to measure the dispersion of a variable. After all, the variance of a variable is equal to the average of the squared deviations from its mean. Thus, the sum of squared errors of prediction is calculated as follows:

$$SS(e) = e'e - \hat{e}'\hat{e} = e'e = \sum e_i^2$$

$$= (-5)^2 + (-5)^2 + (+5)^2 + (+5)^2$$

$$= 25 + 25 + 25 + 25 = 100$$

Note that this equation for the sum of squared errors is simplified by the fact that the mean of the errors is equal to zero.

It turns out that we can obtain a regression equation that minimizes this sum of the squared errors of prediction for a given set of observations. The regression equation that minimizes the sum of the squared errors of prediction is known as the least-squares regression equation. The least-squares regression coefficient for these data is given by:

$$b = 2.5$$

We shall see later how this least-squares regression coefficient was computed. Once the least-squares regression coefficient is computed, the least-squares intercept can be computed as follows:

$$a = \bar{y} - b\bar{x} = 22.5 - (2.5)(15) = -12$$

As before, this equation for the intercept insures that the errors of prediction have a mean of zero.

In order to demonstrate the properties of the least-squares regression coefficient for these data, it is necessary first to compute the predicted scores associated with this regression equation as follows:

$$\hat{\mathbf{y}} \;=\; \mathbf{u}a + \mathbf{x}b \;=\; \begin{bmatrix} 1 \\ 1 \\ 1 \\ 1 \end{bmatrix} (-12) + \begin{bmatrix} 12 \\ 16 \\ 14 \\ 18 \end{bmatrix} 2.5$$

$$= \begin{bmatrix} -12 \\ -12 \\ -12 \\ -12 \end{bmatrix} + \begin{bmatrix} 30 \\ 40 \\ 35 \\ 45 \end{bmatrix} = \begin{bmatrix} 18 \\ 28 \\ 23 \\ 33 \end{bmatrix}$$

The errors of prediction associated with the least-squares regression line are presented in Figure 5.2. At first glance, this least-squares regression line does not appear to be much of an improvement over the arbitrary regression line. It is much closer to some observed values and slightly farther away from others. However, it can be shown that the least-squares regression line does provide a much smaller sum of squared errors of prediction.

We can demonstrate this fact by calculating the errors of prediction associated with the predicted scores produced by this regression equation as follows:

$$\mathbf{e} = \mathbf{y} - \hat{\mathbf{y}} = \begin{bmatrix} 16 \\ 22 \\ 29 \\ 35 \end{bmatrix} - \begin{bmatrix} 18 \\ 28 \\ 23 \\ 33 \end{bmatrix} = \begin{bmatrix} -2 \\ -6 \\ 6 \\ 2 \end{bmatrix}$$

Next, we calculate the sum of squared errors of prediction associated with the least-squares regression equation as follows:

$$SS(e) = \mathbf{e}'\mathbf{e} = \Sigma e_i^2$$

$$= (-2)^2 + (-6)^2 + (6)^2 + (2)^2$$

$$= 4 + 36 + 36 + 4 = 80$$

Given that the sum of squared errors associated with the arbitrary regression equation is equal to 100, it is apparent that the least-squares

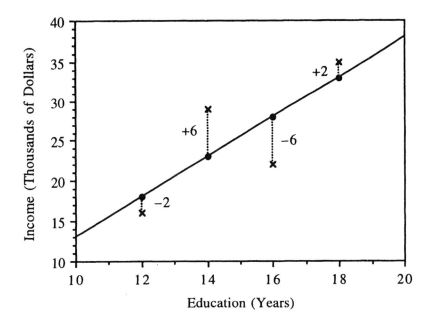

Figure 5.2. Errors of Least-Squares Regression Function

regression equation produces a sum of squared errors that is smaller than the sum of squared errors associated with the arbitrary regression equation. Indeed, it can be proven that there is no other regression equation that can produce a smaller sum of squared errors for these data.

Finally, it is worth noting that this empirical example demonstrates one of the characteristics of the least-squares estimation procedure. As shown in Figure 5.2, the least-squares regression line is closer to the two extreme cases, with respect to both education and income, than it is to the two less extreme cases. As a general rule, the value of the least-squares regression coefficient is greatly influenced by extreme cases. Indeed, the least-squares regression coefficient is "sensitive" to extreme cases, those with either large or small values on both the dependent and independent variables. This property of the least-squares regression coefficient has a certain intuitive appeal. After all, it is the cases with the largest observed values on both the dependent and the independent variables that provide us with most of the information about the exact direction of any relationship between them.

CHAPTER 6

Least-Squares Regression and Covariance

Most of regression analysis is based on least-squares estimates of the parameters of the linear regression equation. Although we have discussed some of the properties of the least-squares regression coefficient already, we have not presented any equations for computing this coefficient. It turns out that the least-squares regression coefficient is based on a quantity known as the covariance. The covariance between two variables is not especially interpretable, but we must become familiar with this quantity because it is central to much of statistical analysis. The generic equation for the covariance between two variables, x and y, is given as follows:

$$\text{Cov}(x, y) \;=\; c_{xy} \;=\; \frac{1}{N} \, (x - \bar{x})'(y - \bar{y})$$

$$= \frac{1}{N} \sum (x_i - \bar{x})(y_i - \bar{y})$$

The covariance between two variables is simply the average product of the values of two variables that have been expressed as deviations from their respective means. It can be seen that this equation bears a striking resemblance to the equation for the variance of a variable. After all, a variance is simply the average squared value of a variable that has been expressed as a deviation from its mean.

As with the equation for the variance of a variable, it is possible to derive a computational form of the equation for the covariance of two variables such that:

$$\text{Cov}(x,y) = \frac{1}{N}(x'y - \bar{x}'\bar{y}) = \frac{1}{N}\sum(x_i y_i - N\bar{x}\bar{y})$$

$$= \frac{1}{N}\sum x_i y_i - \bar{x}\bar{y}$$

This computational equation suggests another interpretation of the covariance of two variables. Specifically, the covariance of two variables is equal to the average product of their respective observed values minus the product of their means. We shall soon see the utility of this interpretation.

In order to see how the covariance between two variables enters into the computation of the least-squares regression coefficient, let us consider the covariance between education, x, and income, y, in the example used earlier such that:

$$\mathbf{x} = \begin{bmatrix} x_1 \\ x_2 \\ x_3 \\ x_4 \end{bmatrix} = \begin{bmatrix} 12 \\ 16 \\ 14 \\ 18 \end{bmatrix} \quad \text{and} \quad \mathbf{y} = \begin{bmatrix} y_1 \\ y_2 \\ y_3 \\ y_4 \end{bmatrix} = \begin{bmatrix} 16 \\ 22 \\ 29 \\ 35 \end{bmatrix}$$

One way to compute the covariance of these two variables is to first compute the scalar product of the vectors of the observed values of the variables as follows:

$$x'y = (12)(16) + (16)(22) + (14)(29) + (18)(35)$$

$$= 192 + 352 + 406 + 630 = 1{,}580$$

This quantity is, of course, simply the sum of the cross products of the respective observed values on these variables. Next, we compute the scalar product of the vectors of the means of these two variables. The computation of this quantity is simplified by the fact that this sum is equal to the number of observations times the product of the two means such that:

$$\bar{x}'\bar{y} \; = \; 4\,(15)(25.5) \; = \; 4\,(382.5) \; = \; 1{,}530$$

Once we have these two quantities, the covariance of variable x and variable y is given by:

$$Cov(x,y) \; = \; \frac{1}{N}\,(x'y - \bar{x}'\bar{y}) \; = \; \frac{1}{4}\,(1{,}580 - 1{,}530)$$

$$= \; \frac{1}{4}\,(50) \; = \; 12.5$$

In other words, the average cross product of education and income, whenever both of these variables are expressed as deviations from their respective means, is 12.5.

The same result can be obtained much more easily by using the computational equation for the covariance as follows:

$$Cov(x,y) \; = \; \frac{1}{N}\sum x_i\,y_i \; - \; \bar{x}\,\bar{y} \; = \; \frac{1}{4}\,(1{,}580) \; - \; (15)(22.5)$$

$$= \; 395 - 382.5 \; = \; 12.5$$

Thus, the average cross product of education and income minus the cross product of their means is 12.5. Aside from these mathematical definitions, the covariance between two variables has no intuitively appealing interpretation. Still, this quantity is important because it enables us to compute the least-squares regression coefficient.

The simple least-squares regression coefficient is equal to the covariance of two variables divided by the variance of the independent variable. The generic formula is given as follows:

$$b_{yx} \; = \; \frac{Cov(x,y)}{Var(x)} \; = \; \frac{c_{xy}}{s_x^2}$$

The proof that this equation yields a regression coefficient that minimizes the sum of the squared errors of prediction requires the use of calculus (see Appendix B). It must be noted that subscripts have been added to this regression coefficient in order to indicate that it represents the regression of variable y on variable x. This notation is sometimes necessary because it is possible to compute a separate regression coefficient for the regression of variable x on variable y. However, these subscripts are often suppressed because it is implicitly assumed, from the context, that variable y is regressed on variable x.

The equation for the least-squares regression coefficient is the ratio of the covariance between the dependent and independent variables to the variance of the independent variable. In this case, the variance of the independent variable, education, can be computed as follows:

$$\mathbf{x'x} = \sum x_i^2 = (12)^2 + (16)^2 + (14)^2 + (18)^2 = 920$$

$$\mathbf{\bar{x}'\bar{x}} = N\bar{x}^2 = 4(15)^2 = 4(225) = 900$$

such that:

$$Var(x) = s_x^2 = \frac{1}{N}(\mathbf{x'x} - \mathbf{\bar{x}'\bar{x}}) = \frac{1}{4}(920 - 900)$$

$$= \frac{1}{4}(20) = 5$$

Of course, the same result can be obtained much more easily by using the computational equation for the variance as follows:

$$Var(x) = \frac{1}{N}\sum x_i^2 - \bar{x}^2 = \frac{1}{4}(920) - (15)^2$$

$$= 230 - 225 = 5$$

Consequently, the least-squares regression coefficient that measures the expected change in variable y, income, associated with a one unit change in variable x, education, is given by:

$$b_{yx} = \frac{Cov(x,y)}{Var(x)} = \frac{c_{xy}}{s_x^2}$$

$$= \frac{12.5}{5.0} = 2.5$$

In short, this regression coefficient suggests that we can expect a 2.5 unit increase in income for every one unit increase in education. More specifically, we can expect income to increase $2,500 for every one year increase in education.

Once we have obtained the least-squares regression coefficient, it is a simple matter to compute the least-squares intercept for this regression equation. As before, the intercept is given by:

$$a_{yx} = \bar{y} - b_{yx}\bar{x}$$

$$= 22.5 - (2.5)(15) = -12$$

Moreover, it can be demonstrated that this equation for the least-squares intercept insures that the regression passes through the means of both variables, as follows:

$$\bar{y} = a_{yx} + b_{yx}\bar{x}$$

$$= -12 + (2.5)(15) = -12 + 37.5 = 22.5$$

In short, the predicted value of variable y for an observation with an average value for variable x is equal to the average value for variable y. As with the regression coefficient, a subscript has been added to the intercept in order to indicate that this is the intercept for the regression of variable y on variable x. This subscript is typically suppressed because it is implicitly assumed that variable y is regressed on variable x.

Finally, it must be noted that the regression coefficient in this particular example had a positive value. However, regression coefficients often have negative values. A negative regression coefficient indicates that there is an inverse relationship between two variables. In other words, an increase in variable x is associated with a decrease in variable y. Moreover, since the variance of a variable is always a positive quantity, the least-squares regression coefficient can assume a negative value only if there is a negative covariance between two variables. A regression coefficient can even have a value of zero. A regression coefficient of zero implies that two variables are linearly independent of one another. In short, a change in variable x does not produce any change in variable y. Since the variance of a variable is always a positive quantity, the least-squares regression coefficient can be zero only if the covariance between two variables is equal to zero.

CHAPTER 7

Covariance and
Linear Independence

Although the covariance between two variables is not immediately interpretable, it is not as esoteric as it might appear at first glance. Indeed, we can understand the concept more clearly if we consider it in the context of the relationship between two binary variables. A binary variable is one that assumes a value of either zero or one. Binary variables are often used to measure simple dichotomies such a gender. For example, we might assign zeros to all the men and ones to all the women. It turns out that the equation for the covariance of two binary variables has a rather simple statistical interpretation. This interpretation obtains for two reasons. First, the mean of a binary variable is equal to its observed probability. Therefore, under the assumption of statistical independence, the product of the means of two binary variables is equal to their expected joint probability. Second, the average cross product of two binary variables is equal to their observed joint probability. Consequently, it can be shown that a covariance of two binary variables measures the extent to which the observed joint distribution of these variables differs from their expected joint distribution under the assumption that they are statistically independent.

We can demonstrate these assertions by examining the components of the equation for the covariance of two variables. Specifically, the computational form of the equation for the covariance of two variables is given by:

$$\text{Cov}(x, y) \;=\; \frac{1}{N}\left(\mathbf{x}'\mathbf{y} - \bar{\mathbf{x}}'\bar{\mathbf{y}}\right) \;=\; \frac{1}{N}\sum x_i\, y_i \;-\; \bar{x}\,\bar{y}$$

It can be shown that the average product of two binary variables is equal to their observed joint probability such that:

$$\frac{1}{N}\sum x_i y_i = P(y=1 \mid x=1)$$

In this equation, the notation $P(y = 1 \mid x = 1)$ refers to the conditional probability that variable y is equal to one given that variable x is equal to one. Similarly, it can be shown that the product of the means of two binary variables is equal to the expected probability that both variable x and variable y are equal to one under the assumption of statistical independence such that:

$$\bar{x}\,\bar{y} = P(y=1)\,P(x=1)$$

In this equation, the notation $P(y = 1)P(x = 1)$ refers to the unconditional probability that variable y is equal to one times the unconditional probability that variable x is equal to one. Consequently, the equation for the covariance of two binary variables is equal to the difference between the observed joint probability of two binary variables and the expected joint probability of those same variables under the assumption of statistical independence such that:

$$\text{Cov}(x,y) = \frac{1}{N}\sum x_i y_i - \bar{x}\,\bar{y}$$

$$= P(y=1 \mid x=1) - P(y=1)\,P(x=1)$$

In order to demonstrate these assertions, let us consider the case of four observations on two binary variables, x and y. To begin with, we might assume that there is no relationship between these two variables. In this case, knowledge of the value of variable x does not enable us to predict the value of variable y. The column vectors for four observations, under this assumption, can be represented as follows:

$$\mathbf{x} = \begin{bmatrix} 1 \\ 1 \\ 0 \\ 0 \end{bmatrix} \quad \text{and} \quad \mathbf{y} = \begin{bmatrix} 1 \\ 0 \\ 1 \\ 0 \end{bmatrix}$$

It can easily be seen that these two binary variables are statistically independent. The likelihood that variable y is equal to one rather than zero is the same whether variable x is equal to one or zero.

It is not difficult to compute the covariance between binary variables because each cross product is either a zero or a one. Using the computational equation, the covariance of these two binary variables can be computed as follows:

$$\text{Cov}(x,y) \;=\; \frac{1}{N}\left(x'y - \bar{x}'\bar{y}\right) \;=\; \frac{1}{N}\sum x_i y_i \;-\; \bar{x}\,\bar{y}$$

$$=\; \frac{1}{4}\,(1) - (0.5)(0.5) \;=\; 0$$

This example demonstrates that the covariance of two statistically independent variables is equal to zero. In other words, variable x and variable y do not covary with one another.

Next, we might assume that two binary variables are perfectly and directly related to one another. In this case, knowledge of the value of variable x enables us to predict exactly the value of variable y. The column vectors for four observations, under this assumption, can be represented as follows:

$$\mathbf{x} \;=\; \begin{bmatrix} 1 \\ 1 \\ 0 \\ 0 \end{bmatrix} \quad \text{and} \quad \mathbf{y} \;=\; \begin{bmatrix} 1 \\ 1 \\ 0 \\ 0 \end{bmatrix}$$

In short, whenever variable x is equal to one, variable y is also equal to one. Conversely, whenever variable x is equal to zero, variable y is also equal to zero.

Using the computational equation once again, the covariance of these two binary variables can be computed as follows:

$$\text{Cov}(x,y) \;=\; \frac{1}{N}\left(x'y - \bar{x}'\bar{y}\right) \;=\; \frac{1}{N}\sum x_i y_i \;-\; \bar{x}\,\bar{y}$$

$$=\; \frac{1}{4}\,(2) - (0.5)(0.5) \;=\; 0.25$$

At first glance, a covariance of 0.25 may not seem very impressive. However, this quantity is more impressive if we note that the variances of both variable x and variable y are also equal to 0.25. The fact that the covariance between two variables is equal to the variance of the independent variable means that the regression coefficient will be equal to one, implying that variable y increases one unit with every one unit increase in variable x.

Finally, we might assume that two binary variables are perfectly but inversely related to one another. In the case of binary variables, an inverse relationship implies that whenever variable x is equal to one, variable y is equal to zero and vice versa. The column vectors for these four observations, under this assumption, can be represented as follows:

$$\mathbf{x} = \begin{bmatrix} 1 \\ 1 \\ 0 \\ 0 \end{bmatrix} \quad \text{and} \quad \mathbf{y} = \begin{bmatrix} 0 \\ 0 \\ 1 \\ 1 \end{bmatrix}$$

Even though this is an inverse relationship, it is still possible to predict the value of the y variable exactly from the value of the x variable. Whenever variable x is equal to one, variable y is equal to zero. Conversely, whenever variable x is equal to zero, variable y is equal to one.

Using the computational equation once again, the covariance of these two binary variables can be computed as follows:

$$\text{Cov}(x,y) = \frac{1}{N}\left(\mathbf{x'y} - \mathbf{\bar{x}'\bar{y}}\right) = \frac{1}{N}\sum x_i y_i - \bar{x}\,\bar{y}$$

$$= \frac{1}{4}(0) - (0.5)(0.5) = -0.25$$

In absolute terms, the magnitude of the covariance between the inversely related variables is equal to the covariance between the directly related variables. However, in the case of an inverse relationship, the covariance is negative. Whenever the covariance between two variables is negative, the regression coefficient between these variables will also be negative, implying that variable y decreases as variable x increases. In this particular case, variable y will decrease one unit with every one unit increase in variable x.

Finally, it must be noted that, in these simple examples, the fact that the covariance between two binary variables is equal to zero implies that these two variables are statistically independent. It is important to understand that a covariance of zero between two variables does not, in general, mean that they are statistically independent. We obtained these results because we were dealing with binary variables. In most cases, of course, we are interested in the covariance between two continuous variables. A covariance of zero between two continuous variables implies only that these variables are linearly independent. *Two variables are linearly independent whenever there is no linear relationship between them.* In short, two variables are linearly independent whenever it is not possible to predict the values of one variable using a linear function of the other variable. It is possible for two variables to be linearly independent even thought there is a perfect curvilinear relationship between them. In this case, the two variables are linearly independent but certainly not statistically independent. Therefore, in regression analysis, we cannot assume that there is no statistical relationship between two variables simply because the regression coefficient between these variables is equal to zero. We can assume only that there is no linear relationship between these variables. There is always the possibility that the relationship between these two variables can be described using a complex mathematical function.

CHAPTER 8

Separating Explained
and Error Variance

In simple regression analysis, we begin with two variables: an independent variable, x, and a dependent variable, y. In the course of the analysis, however, we create two new variables. One of these variables, $\hat{y}$, is the predicted value of the dependent variable using the linear regression equation and the independent variable. The other variable, e, is the error of prediction obtained using this regression equation. This error value is sometimes referred to as a residual value because it is simply the difference between the observed y value and the predicted y value. These two variables, the predicted value of the dependent variable, $\hat{y}$, and the error of prediction, e, are defined mathematically, in vector notation, as follows:

$$\hat{y} = ua + xb$$

$$e = y - \hat{y}$$

It has already been noted that the errors of prediction are very important in regression analysis because they tell us how well the model "fits" the data. It will also be recalled that the objective of least-squares regression is to obtain a regression coefficient and an intercept that minimize the sum of the squared errors of prediction and, therefore, the variance of these errors.

One of the most important and useful properties of regression analysis is that it permits us to partition the observed or "total" variance in the dependent variable into two separate components:

"explained" variance and "error" variance. We begin with the equation for the observed values on the dependent variable expressed as the sum of the predicted values and the errors of prediction as follows:

$$\mathbf{y} = \hat{\mathbf{y}} + \mathbf{e}$$

Given this equation, it is possible to decompose the inner product of the vector of observed values into several different components such that:

$$
\begin{aligned}
\mathbf{y'y} &= (\hat{\mathbf{y}} + \mathbf{e})'(\hat{\mathbf{y}} + \mathbf{e}) \\
&= \hat{\mathbf{y}}'(\hat{\mathbf{y}} + \mathbf{e}) + \mathbf{e}'(\hat{\mathbf{y}} + \mathbf{e}) \\
&= \hat{\mathbf{y}}'\hat{\mathbf{y}} + \hat{\mathbf{y}}'\mathbf{e} + \mathbf{e}'\hat{\mathbf{y}} + \mathbf{e}'\mathbf{e}
\end{aligned}
$$

It turns out that this equation can be simplified by the fact that two of these quantities, $\hat{\mathbf{y}}'\mathbf{e}$ and $\mathbf{e}'\hat{\mathbf{y}}$, are equal to zero. This result is important because it insures that the covariance between the predicted y values and the errors of prediction is equal to zero such that:

$$\text{Cov}(\hat{\mathbf{y}}, \mathbf{e}) = \frac{1}{N}(\hat{\mathbf{y}}'\mathbf{e}) = 0$$

The proof of this result is too complicated to present at this point, but we can demonstrate it later.

Therefore, the sum of squares of the dependent variable is equal to the sum of squares of the predicted values plus the sum of squares of the errors of prediction such that:

$$
\begin{aligned}
\text{SS(y)} = \mathbf{y'y} &= \hat{\mathbf{y}}'\hat{\mathbf{y}} + \mathbf{e}'\mathbf{e} \\
&= \text{SS}(\hat{y}) + \text{SS}(e)
\end{aligned}
$$

Consequently, the variance of the dependent variable is equal to the sum of the variance of the predicted values and the variance of the errors of prediction as follows:

$$\text{Var(y)} = \frac{1}{N}\text{SS(y)} = \frac{1}{N}\text{SS}(\hat{y}) + \frac{1}{N}\text{SS}(e)$$

$$= \text{Var}(\hat{y}) + \text{Var}(e)$$

In other words, the "total" variance in the dependent variable can be partitioned into two parts: "explained" variance and "error" variance.

These results can be demonstrated using the example of the relationship between education and income among four individuals. The predicted income values obtained using the least-squares regression equation and the observed education values are as follows:

$$\hat{y} = \mathbf{u}a + \mathbf{x}b = \mathbf{u}(-12) + \mathbf{x}(2.5)$$

$$= \begin{bmatrix} 1 \\ 1 \\ 1 \\ 1 \end{bmatrix} (-12) + \begin{bmatrix} 12 \\ 16 \\ 14 \\ 18 \end{bmatrix} (2.5)$$

$$= \begin{bmatrix} -12 \\ -12 \\ -12 \\ -12 \end{bmatrix} + \begin{bmatrix} 30 \\ 40 \\ 35 \\ 45 \end{bmatrix} = \begin{bmatrix} 18 \\ 28 \\ 23 \\ 33 \end{bmatrix}$$

Similarly, the errors of prediction obtained using these predicted values are as follows:

$$\mathbf{e} = \mathbf{y} - \hat{\mathbf{y}} = \begin{bmatrix} 16 \\ 22 \\ 29 \\ 35 \end{bmatrix} - \begin{bmatrix} 18 \\ 28 \\ 23 \\ 33 \end{bmatrix} = \begin{bmatrix} -2 \\ -6 \\ 6 \\ 2 \end{bmatrix}$$

Given that the mean of the predicted values of the dependent variable is equal to the mean of the observed values of the dependent variable, the variance of the predicted values can be readily obtained as follows:·

$$\text{Var}(\hat{y}) = \frac{1}{N} (\hat{\mathbf{y}}'\hat{\mathbf{y}} - \bar{\mathbf{y}}'\bar{\mathbf{y}}) = \frac{1}{N} \sum \hat{y}_i^2 - \bar{y}^2$$

$$= \frac{1}{4}(2726) - (25.5)^2$$

$$= 681.50 - 650.25 = 31.25$$

Similarly, given that the mean of the errors of prediction is equal to zero, the variance of the errors of prediction can be obtained as follows:

$$\text{Var}(e) = \frac{1}{N}(e'e - \bar{e}'\bar{e}) = \frac{1}{N}(e'e) = \frac{1}{N}\sum e_i^2$$

$$= \frac{1}{4}(80) = 20$$

We have already indicated that the variance of the dependent variable is equal to the sum of the variance of the predicted values and the variance of the errors of prediction. This can be demonstrated as follows:

$$\text{Var}(y) = \frac{1}{N}(y'y - \bar{y}'\bar{y}) = \frac{1}{N}\sum y_i^2 - \bar{y}^2$$

$$= \frac{1}{4}(2,806) - (25.5)^2$$

$$= 701.50 - 650.25 = 51.25$$

such that:

$$\text{Var}(y) = \text{Var}(\hat{y}) + \text{Var}(e) = 31.25 + 20.00 = 51.25$$

Finally, given this decomposition of total variance into explained variance and error variance, we can determine the proportion of the variance in the observed y variable that is attributable to or explained by the linear regression equation using the observed x variable. This ratio forms the basis of a statistic known as the "coefficient of determination." *The coefficient of determination measures the proportion of the variance in the dependent variable that is accounted for by the independent variable.* This quantity is also referred to as the "r-square" of a regression equation. There are a number of different equations for computing the coefficient of determination. For example, one equation expresses this coefficient as the ratio of the variance of the predicted values to the variance of the observed values of the dependent variable as follows:

$$r_{yx}^2 = \frac{\text{Var}(\hat{y})}{\text{Var}(y)}$$

$$= \frac{31.25}{51.25} = 0.61$$

Alternatively, the equation for the coefficient of determination is sometimes expressed in terms of the quantity one minus the ratio of error variance to observed variance as follows:

$$r_{yx}^2 = 1 - \left(\frac{\text{Var}(e)}{\text{Var}(y)} \right)$$

$$= 1 - \left(\frac{20.00}{51.25} \right) = 1 - 0.39 = 0.61$$

Using either of these equations for the coefficient of determination, it is apparent that 61 percent of the variance in income can be "explained" or "accounted for" by the least-squares regression equation using education as the independent variable.

The coefficient of determination is known as a "goodness of fit" statistic because it tells us how well a given regression model "fits" the data. Specifically, the coefficient of determination ranges in value from zero to a positive one. For example, whenever there is no relationship between the dependent variable and the independent variable, the variance of the errors of prediction will be equal to the variance of the dependent variable. In this case, the coefficient of determination will be equal to zero. Conversely, whenever there is an exact linear relationship between the dependent variable and the independent variable, the variance of the errors of prediction will be equal to zero. In this case, the coefficient of determination will be equal to one. This statistic is very useful because it enables us to compare different independent variables in order to determine which one is "best" in terms of explaining the variance in the dependent variable.

CHAPTER 9

Transforming Variables to Standard Form

There are occasions when it is desirable to convert a variable into a more convenient form by standardizing it. *A standardized variable is one that has been transformed so that it has a mean of zero and a variance of one.* Standardization can be very useful because it enables us to compare the regression of a dependent variable on different independent variables. It is much easier to compare the relative magnitudes of different regression coefficients if the variables have the same variances. For example, it is difficult to compare the regression of income on education with the regression of income on occupational prestige because the differences in the regression coefficients for these two independent variables are attributable, at least in part, to the fact that they have different variances. By converting both of these independent variables to standard form, we can compare the change in income we expect with a one standard deviation change in education to the change in income we expect with a one standard deviation change in occupational prestige.

The first step in standardizing a variable involves expressing each observed value as a deviation from the mean for that variable. These values are sometimes referred to as the mean deviation values of a variable. Specifically, the mean deviation values for a variable are given by:

$$d = x - \bar{x}$$

One of the most important properties of any variable in mean deviation form is that it has a mean of zero such that:

$$\text{Mean}(d) = \frac{1}{N} \mathbf{u}'\mathbf{d} = \frac{1}{N} \sum d_i = 0$$

However, the transformation of a variable to mean deviation form does not alter its variance such that:

$$\text{Var}(d) = \frac{1}{N}(\mathbf{d}'\mathbf{d} - \overline{\mathbf{d}}'\overline{\mathbf{d}}) = \frac{1}{N}\mathbf{d}'\mathbf{d}$$

$$= \frac{1}{N}(\mathbf{x} - \overline{\mathbf{x}})'(\mathbf{x} - \overline{\mathbf{x}}) = \text{Var}(x)$$

In short, since the variance of a variable is equal to the average of the squared deviations from its mean, the variance of a variable is not affected by the transformation to mean deviation form.

It might be noted that it is possible to conduct a regression analysis in which both the dependent and independent variables have been transformed to mean deviation form. One advantage of conducting a regression analysis with variables in mean deviation form is that the regression equation does not include an intercept. Specifically, it can be demonstrated that the intercept of a regression equation is equal to zero whenever both the dependent and the independent variables have means of zero as follows:

$$a = \overline{y} - b_{yx}\overline{x}$$

$$= 0 - b_{yx}0 = 0$$

Although they are relatively rare, there are situations in which we might be interested in the regression of one variable on another given that both variables are expressed as deviations from their respective means.

The second step in standardizing a variable involves dividing each mean deviation value by the standard deviation of that variable. *The standard deviation of a variable is equal to the square root of its variance.* Specifically, the equation for the standard deviation of a variable is given by:

$$s = \sqrt{\text{Var}(x)} = \sqrt{s^2}$$

The standard deviation is an alternative measure of the dispersion of a variable. Given that the variance of a variable is equal to the average of the squared deviations from its mean, the variance is invariably much larger than the average absolute deviation from the mean. Therefore, the variance is not a very intuitively appealing measure of dispersion. The standard deviation is more appealing as a measure of dispersion simply because it is more directly comparable to the average absolute deviation from the mean.

Once we have obtained the standard deviation of a variable, we can obtain the standardized values of that variable simply by dividing the mean deviation values by their standard deviation. The equation for these standardized values, which are often referred to as "z scores," is given as follows:

$$z = \frac{1}{s} d = \frac{1}{s} (x - \bar{x})$$

In standard notation, each z value is given by the following equation:

$$z_i = \frac{d_i}{s} = \frac{x_i - \bar{x}}{s}$$

We can demonstrate the necessary calculations using the earlier example of the educations, in years of schooling, of four individuals such that:

$$x = \begin{bmatrix} 12 \\ 16 \\ 14 \\ 18 \end{bmatrix}$$

It will be recalled that the mean and variance of this variable were given earlier as follows:

$$\text{Mean}(x) = \bar{x} = 15$$

$$\text{Var}(x) = s^2 = 5$$

Consequently, the standard deviation of this variable can be obtained by simply computing the square root of its variance such that:

$$\text{S.D.}(x) = s = \sqrt{s^2}$$

$$= \sqrt{5} = 2.24$$

In order to obtain the standardized values for a variable, we must first compute each of the mean deviation values as follows:

$$\mathbf{d} = \mathbf{x} - \bar{\mathbf{x}}$$

$$= \begin{bmatrix} 12 - 15 \\ 16 - 15 \\ 14 - 15 \\ 18 - 15 \end{bmatrix} = \begin{bmatrix} -3 \\ 1 \\ -1 \\ 3 \end{bmatrix}$$

Next, we divide each of these mean deviation values by the standard deviation to obtain the standardized values as follows:

$$\mathbf{z} = \frac{1}{s}(\mathbf{x} - \bar{\mathbf{x}}) = \frac{1}{s}\mathbf{d}$$

$$= \frac{1}{2.24}\begin{bmatrix} -3 \\ 1 \\ -1 \\ 3 \end{bmatrix} = \begin{bmatrix} -1.34 \\ 0.45 \\ -0.45 \\ 1.34 \end{bmatrix}$$

It can be verified that this standardized variable has a mean of zero as follows:

$$\text{Mean}(z) = \bar{z} = \frac{1}{N}\mathbf{u}'\mathbf{z} = \frac{1}{N}\sum z_i$$

$$= \frac{1}{4} (-1.34 + 0.45 - 0.45 + 1.34) \quad = \frac{1}{4} (0) = 0$$

Similarly, it can also be verified that this standardized variable has a variance of one as follows:

$$\text{Var}(z) = s^2 = \frac{1}{N} \mathbf{z'z} = \frac{1}{N} \sum z_i^2$$

$$= \frac{1}{4} (1.80 + 0.20 + 0.20 + 1.80) = \frac{1}{4} (4) = 1$$

As we shall see, standardized variables are often very useful in regression analysis precisely because they have the same variance, which is easy to interpret because it is equal to one.

CHAPTER 10

Regression Analysis with Standardized Variables

The standardization of both the dependent and independent variables in regression analysis leads to a number of important results. To begin with, the regression coefficient between two standardized variables is equal to the covariance of the standardized variables. This result can be seen from the following equation for the regression coefficient:

$$b_{yx}^* = \frac{\text{Cov}(z_y, z_x)}{\text{Var}(z_x)} = \frac{\text{Cov}(z_y, z_x)}{1} = \text{Cov}(z_y, z_x)$$

In order to avoid confusion, the standardized regression coefficient, b_{yx}^*, is denoted with an asterisk in order to distinguish it from the unstandardized regression coefficient, b_{yx}. Moreover, the standardized regression coefficient for the regression of variable y on variable x is equal to the standardized regression coefficient for the regression of variable x on variable y such that:

$$b_{yx}^* = b_{xy}^*$$

These two standardized regression coefficients are equal to one another because the covariances in their numerators are the same and the variances in their denominators are both equal to one.

We can demonstrate the calculations required to obtain the standardized regression coefficient using, once again, the example of the regression of income on education for four individuals. The standard scores for both variable x, education, and variable y, income, are given as follows:

$$z_x = \frac{1}{s_x}(x - \bar{x}) = \frac{1}{2.24}\begin{bmatrix} 12 - 15 \\ 16 - 15 \\ 14 - 15 \\ 18 - 15 \end{bmatrix} = \begin{bmatrix} -1.34 \\ 0.45 \\ -0.45 \\ 1.34 \end{bmatrix}$$

and

$$z_y = \frac{1}{s_y}(y - \bar{y}) = \frac{1}{7.16}\begin{bmatrix} 16 - 25.5 \\ 22 - 25.5 \\ 27 - 25.5 \\ 35 - 25.5 \end{bmatrix} = \begin{bmatrix} -1.33 \\ -0.49 \\ 0.49 \\ 1.33 \end{bmatrix}$$

Given the fact that these standardized scores have means that are equal to zero, their covariance is simply the average product of their respective standardized scores as follows:

$$\begin{aligned} \text{Cov}(z_y, z_x) &= \frac{1}{N} z_y' z_x = \frac{1}{N}\sum z_{yi} z_{xi} \\ &= \frac{1}{4}(1.78 - 0.22 - 0.22 + 1.78) \\ &= \frac{1}{4}(3.12) = 0.78 \end{aligned}$$

This covariance between the two variables in standard form is equal, of course, to the standardized regression coefficient between them.

Fortunately, it is not necessary to compute standardized scores in order to calculate the standardized regression coefficient between two variables. Instead, it is possible to obtain the standardized regression coefficient directly from the unstandardized regression coefficient using the following equation:

$$b_{yx}^{*} = b_{yx} \left(\frac{s_x}{s_y} \right)$$

In short, we can obtain the standardized regression coefficient, b_{yx}^{*}, by multiplying the unstandardized regression coefficient, b_{yx}, by the ratio of the standard deviation of the independent variable to the standard deviation of the dependent variable.

This result can also be verified using this same example. It will be recalled, for example, that the unstandardized regression coefficient for the regression of income on education and the variances of these two variables were given as follows:

$$b_{yx} = 2.5$$

$$s_x^2 = 5.00$$

$$s_y^2 = 51.25$$

Of course, the standard deviations of both variables can be obtained simply by calculating the square roots of their variances as follows:

$$\text{S.D.}(x) = s_x = \sqrt{s_x^2} = \sqrt{5.00} = 2.239$$

$$\text{S.D.}(y) = s_y = \sqrt{s_y^2} = \sqrt{51.25} = 7.159$$

Therefore, it is possible to obtain the corresponding standardized regression coefficient between these two variables as follows:

$$b_{yx}^{*} = b_{yx} \left(\frac{s_x}{s_y} \right) = 2.5 \left(\frac{2.236}{7.159} \right)$$

$$= 2.5 \, (0.312) = 0.78$$

In short, we do not need to conduct any special analyses in order to obtain the standardized regression coefficient between two variables.

It is worth noting that the interpretation of a standardized regression coefficient differs somewhat from that of an unstandardized regression coefficient.   An unstandardized regression coefficient measures the expected change in the dependent variable associated with a one unit change in the independent variable.   Therefore, the standardized regression coefficient measures the expected standard deviation change in the dependent variable associated with a one standard deviation change in the independent variable.   This interpretation follows directly from the equation for the predicted value of the dependent variable with both variables in standard form.   In this case, this predication is given by:

$$\hat{z}_y = z_x b_{yx}^* = z_x (0.78)$$

It will be noted that this equation does not include an intercept because the dependent and independent variables have means of zero.

In this particular example, a one standard deviation increase in education can be expected to produce a 0.78 standard deviation increase in income.   This interpretation of the standardized regression coefficient can prove to be very useful whenever we wish to compare the standardized regression coefficients for different independent variables with respect to the same dependent variable.   Moreover, whenever we know the standard deviations of the variables, we can easily convert the results of the regression analysis with standardized variables into the corresponding results of a regression analysis with unstandardized variables.   For example, given the standardized regression coefficient and the standard deviation of the dependent variable, we can calculate the increase in income, in dollars, associated with a one standard deviation increase in education as follows:

$$\Delta y = b_{yx}^* s_y = (0.78)(7.159) = 5.584$$

In other words, given the fact that the standard deviation of income is $7,159, we expect a change that is equal to only 0.78 of this standard deviation, or $5,584, for every one standard deviation increase in education.   We can obtain roughly the same results using the unstandardized regression coefficient and the standard deviation of the independent variable as follows:

$$\Delta y = b_{yx} s_x = (2.5)(2.236) = 5.590$$

Since we expect income to increase $2,500 for every one year increase in education, we must expect income to increase by $5,590 with an increase in education of 2.236 years. The slight difference in the results obtained using these two approaches is attributable to rounding error.

Moreover, it must be pointed out that regression analysis has a special term for the covariance between two standardized variables. *The covariance between two standardized variables is equal to the correlation between these variables.* This interpretation of correlation can be demonstrated using the standard equation for the correlation coefficient as the covariance between two variables divided by the product of their standard deviations. Since the standard deviation of a standardized variable is equal to one, the correlation coefficient between two variables is equal to the covariance of these variables in standard form such that:

$$r_{yx} = \frac{\mathrm{Cov}(y,x)}{\mathrm{S.D.}(y)\,\mathrm{S.D.}(x)} = \frac{\mathrm{Cov}(z_y,z_x)}{\mathrm{S.D.}(z_y)\,\mathrm{S.D.}(z_x)}$$

$$= \frac{\mathrm{Cov}(z_y,z_x)}{1} = \mathrm{Cov}(z_y,z_x)$$

This implies, of course, that the correlation coefficient and the two standardized regression coefficients are equal to one another such that:

$$r_{yx} = r_{xy} = b^*_{yx} = b^*_{xy}$$

It can be demonstrated that the absolute value of the correlation coefficient and the two standardized regression coefficients cannot exceed one. In other words, these coefficients always range in value from a negative one to a positive one. A correlation coefficient will be equal to either a positive one or a negative one only if there is a perfect linear relationship between two variables. In this case, the coefficient of determination, which is equal to the square of the correlation coefficient, will also be equal to one. Conversely, a correlation coefficient will be equal to zero only if there is no linear relationship at all between two variables. In this case, of course, the coefficient of determination will also be equal to zero.

CHAPTER 11

Populations, Samples, and Sampling Distributions

To this point, we have used regression analysis only to describe the relationship between two variables in a sample. However, in statistical analysis, we are not usually interested in the characteristics of a particular sample. More often, we are interested in estimating the characteristics of the population from which the sample was drawn. Whenever we wish to make statements about the characteristics of a population, based on the characteristics of a sample, we must rely on the logic of statistical inference. In particular, we must employ the concept of sampling distributions. Indeed, the logic of inferential statistics is based largely on the concept of sampling distributions. *A sampling distribution is the theoretical distribution of a sample statistic that would be obtained from a large number of random samples of equal size from a population.* Consequently, the sampling distribution serves as a statistical "bridge" between a known sample and the unknown population. Sample statistics, such as the sample mean and variance, are used to provide estimates of corresponding population parameters, such as the population mean and variance.

In order to understand the process of statistical inference more clearly, let us consider the sampling distribution of the simplest of all sample statistics: the mean. If we take more than one sample from the same population and compute a mean for each sample, we are likely to discover that the sample means are not equal to one another. Each mean is slightly different because each one describes a sample composed, by and large, of different observations. We explain the fact that different samples from the same population yield different sample statistics in terms of sampling error. For example, let us assume that we wish to estimate the average family income in the United States. This statistic is known as a population parameter because it describes the mean of the income distribution in the population. In order to get an accurate estimate of this population parameter, we might take a large number of random samples of the same size from this population. A sample is referred to as random if every member of the population has an equal chance of being included in the sample. If we compute the mean family income for each of these samples, we will almost certainly end up with a number of different estimates of the average family income in the population. Indeed, we will discover that we have a distribution of sample means. Some means will be more frequent than others. There will be relatively few small means and relatively few large means. Most of the sample means will cluster around an average value.

It can be shown that the distribution of all these sample means will approximate a normal distribution. This is an important result because the normal distribution is a theoretical distribution that can be described precisely by a mathematical function. Indeed, the normal distribution was invented by statisticians. The fact that the distribution of the means from a large number of samples of equal size from a population approximates a normal distribution is a result of the *central limit theorem*. This theorem is one of the most powerful results in all of statistical analysis. Perhaps the most remarkable property of this theorem is that the sampling distribution of the mean of a variable will approximate a normal distribution even if the distribution of that variable in the population is not normal. For example, the distribution of family income in America is hardly normal. To the contrary, it is a highly skewed distribution inasmuch as there are millions of very poor families and only a few hundred very rich families in the population. Nevertheless, the central limit theorem assures us that the sampling distribution of the mean for this variable approximates a normal distribution. In other words, there will be only a few samples in which the average income is either very small or very large. Most of the samples will have average incomes that cluster around a central value.

Normal distributions come in many different shapes. Indeed, a normal distribution can have any mean and any finite variance. Fortunately, the central limit theorem specifies both the mean and the variance of the sampling distribution of the mean. To begin with, it states that the mean of the sampling distribution of the mean is equal to population mean such that:

$$\text{Mean}(\bar{x}) = \mu_x$$

Statisticians typically refer to population parameters with Greek letters. In this case, the population mean is represented by the Greek letter mu, μ. The fact that the mean of the sampling distribution of the mean is equal to the population mean assures us that the sample mean provides an unbiased estimate of the population mean. In short, the sample mean is, on average, equal to the population mean. In addition, the central limit theorem states that the standard deviation of the sampling distribution of the mean is equal to the standard deviation of the population divided by the square root of the sample size such that:

$$\text{S.D.}(\bar{x}) = \frac{\sigma_x}{\sqrt{N}} = \sigma_{\bar{x}}$$

In this case, the population standard deviation is represented by the Greek letter sigma, σ. *In statistics, the standard deviation of a sampling distribution of any statistic is called its standard error.* This standard error tells us how much variation there is among the different sample means. As a rule, we want our sample statistics to have relatively small standard errors because they provide more accurate estimates of the associated population parameters.

As this equation indicates, the standard error of the mean depends on two separate quantities: the standard deviation of the variable in the population and the size of the sample. The standard error of the mean will decrease with decreases in the standard deviation of the variable in the population. This result makes a great deal of sense. If there is very little variation in the population, there will be very little variation in each sample and very little variation among the means of different samples. Conversely, if there is a great deal of variation in the population, there is likely to be a great deal of variation in the sample means. Moreover, the standard error of the mean will decrease with increases in sample size. Specifically, there is an exponential relationship between sample size and the standard error of the mean. If we wish to reduce the standard error of the mean by half, we must quadruple the size of the sample. We can also demonstrate that, as sample size approaches infinity, the standard error of the mean approaches zero. This result makes a great deal of sense. If the samples include almost the entire population, there will be very little variation in the means of these samples.

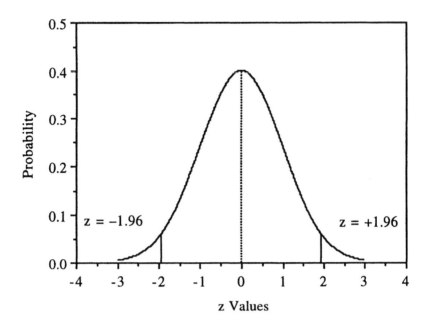

Figure 11.1. Normal Distribution and Critical z Values

The fact that the sampling distribution of the mean is approximately normal whenever sample size is large is important because we know a great deal about the normal distribution. Given that the normal distribution is literally defined by a precise mathematical function, we can calculate the proportion of the area under this curve between any two points. This result is very useful because we can equate area to probability. For example, we know that exactly 95 percent of the total area under the curve for a normal distribution is within 1.96 standard deviations of the mean of this distribution. By equating area to probability, we can say that 95 percent of all possible sample means are within 1.96 standard errors of the population mean. Stated somewhat differently, we can say that there is only a 5 percent chance that any sample mean is more than 1.96 standard errors from the population mean. A graph of the normal distribution and the area associated with 1.96 standard errors above and below the mean is presented in Figure 11.1. The importance of the sampling distribution is that it enables us to calculate the probability of a particular sample statistic. For example, if we know the population mean and standard deviation of a variable in the population, we can calculate the probability of obtaining any given sample mean. If a sample mean is more than 1.96 standard errors larger or smaller than the population mean, we can state that there is no more than a 5 percent probability that the sample came from this population.

Finally, it must be reiterated that the central limit theorem is based on the assumption of large sample sizes. Indeed, the sampling distribution of the mean will be exactly normal only in the case of infinitely large samples. However, the sampling distribution of the mean will begin to approximate a normal distribution, regardless of the population distribution, whenever we have samples with a few hundred cases. Conversely, the sampling distribution of the mean will approximate a normal distribution, even in very small samples, if the variable has a normal distribution in the population. Fortunately, statisticians have established that the central limit theorem is very robust in the sense that the results of this theorem obtain even when some of its assumptions have not been met. For example, we know that the sampling distribution of the mean will be approximately normal, even in relatively small samples, whenever the distribution of a variable in the population has a relatively symmetric and unimodal distribution.

CHAPTER 12

Sampling Distributions and Test Statistics

The fact that the sampling distribution of the mean approximates a normal distribution, which can be described exactly by a mathematical function, enables us to test certain hypotheses using statistical inference. In statistical inference, we make an assumption about a population parameter and then determine whether or not our sample statistics are consistent with that assumption, allowing for the effects of sampling error. The assumption that we wish to test is usually referred to as the *null hypothesis*. For example, we might want to determine whether or not the average family income of a particular minority group is equal to the average family income of the population as a whole. For the purposes of this example, we will assume that we know both the mean and the standard deviation of the distribution of family income in the population. Specifically, we shall assume that the population mean is $24,000 and that the population standard deviation is $2,000. In order to test this hypothesis, we will also assume that we have randomly sampled 1,600 minority group families and have found that their average family income is $23,900. The question that we want to answer is whether or not the difference between the sample mean and population mean can be attributed to sampling error or represents a real difference between the minority group and the population.

In the jargon of statistical inference, we wish to test the null hypothesis that the average family income of the minority group, as measured by the sample mean, is equal to the average family income of the population as a whole, as measured by the population mean. In other words, the null hypothesis asserts that there is no difference between the minority group and the population with respect to income. It is customary to state such a null hypothesis symbolically as follows:

$$H_0 : \overline{x} = \mu_x$$

In statistical inference, we test a null hypothesis and either reject it or fail to reject it. If we fail to reject this null hypothesis, then we infer that the average family income of the minority group is equal to the average family income in the population. Conversely, if we reject this null hypothesis, then we infer that the average family income of the minority group is not equal to the average family income in the population.

In this particular example, we want to determine whether or not the $100 difference between the population mean and the sample mean is statistically significant in the sense that it cannot be attributed to sampling error. In effect, we wish to rule out sampling error as a likely explanation for this observed difference in the two means. Before we can answer this question, however, we must specify what we mean by "likely." By convention, statisticians typically assume that a difference between a population parameter and a sample statistic is "statistically significant" if it could have occurred by chance in only 5 out of every 100 samples as a result of sampling error. Once we have established such a significance level, we can examine the sampling distribution of our statistic to determine whether or not we can reject the null hypothesis.

The central limit theorem assures us that the distribution of the sample mean will approximate a normal distribution. Moreover, the cumulative probability density function for the normal distribution tells us that, in 95 out of 100 samples, the sample mean will be within 1.96 standard errors of the population mean. We can compute the standard error of the sample mean as follows:

$$\sigma_{\overline{x}} = \frac{\sigma_x}{\sqrt{N}} = \frac{2,000}{\sqrt{1,600}}$$

$$= \frac{2,000}{40} = 50$$

Consequently, we can compute the range of sample means that must lie within 1.96 standard errors of the mean of the sampling distribution as follows:

$$(\pm 1.96)(\sigma_{\bar{x}}) = (\pm 1.96)(50) = \pm 98$$

Given a population with this mean and standard deviation, 95 out of every 100 samples of this size will have means that range between $23,902 and $24,098. Conversely, only 5 out of every 100 samples of this size will have means smaller than $23,902 or larger than $24,908 as the result of sampling error. Consequently, a difference of means greater than $98 can be attributed to sampling error no more than 5 percent of the time. In this example, we reject the null hypothesis that the sample mean is equal to the population mean and infer that the mean family income of this minority group is not equal to the mean family income of the population at large.

A simpler way of approaching this problem is to employ a test statistic. *A test statistic is any statistic that is calculated for the sole purpose of testing a hypothesis.* Typically, test statistics are mathematical functions of sample statistics. In this particular case, we can compute a z statistic. Specifically, we transform the mean for the minority group into a standardized value. First, we subtract the mean of the sampling distribution, which is equal to the population mean, from the mean of our sample. Second, we divide this mean deviation value by the standard deviation of the sampling distribution. The result is a z value given by:

$$z_{\bar{x}} = \frac{\bar{x} - \mu_x}{\sigma_{\bar{x}}}$$

This standardization has the effect of transforming all of the sample means into a deviation from a mean of zero in a distribution with a standard deviation of one. In short, we have transformed the sampling distribution of the mean, which was a normal distribution with a mean of $24,000 and a standard deviation of 50, into a standard normal distribution with a mean of zero and a standard deviation of one. The transformation of a sampling distribution into standard form enables us to compute the probability associated with any deviation from the mean of this distribution. Therefore, once we have calculated this test statistic, we can evaluate it with respect to the cumulative probability density function of the standard normal distribution.

We can illustrate the utility of the z statistic as a test statistic using the same example involving the average income of a minority group and the average income of the population as a whole. Given the standard error of the mean as before, we can compute the z statistic for this sample mean as follows:

$$z_{\bar{x}} = \frac{\bar{x} - \mu_x}{\sigma_{\bar{x}}} = \frac{23,900 - 24,000}{50}$$

$$= \frac{-100}{50} = -2.0$$

This test statistic tells us that our observed sample mean is two standard errors below the mean of the sampling distribution. In order to assess the statistical significance of this test statistic, we must refer to a table of critical values for the standard normal distribution. Such a table tells us the value of the z statistic associated with each possible probability level. These probability levels are also called *critical regions* because they refer to those regions near the tails of the normal distribution that are associated with statistically significant deviations from the mean. Based on our knowledge of the critical regions for the standard normal distribution, we know that only 5 percent of the area under the standard normal curve is more than 1.96 standard deviations above or below the mean of zero under the null hypothesis. This implies that the probability of obtaining a sample mean which yields a z statistic smaller than −1.96 or greater than +1.96 under the null hypothesis is no more than 5 percent. Since our z test value exceeds the critical value of 1.96 associated with the 0.05 probability level, we reject the null hypothesis. In short, we infer that the difference in average family incomes between the minority group and the population at large is statistically significant.

In this example, we have assumed that it was appropriate to test the null hypothesis using the conventional 0.05 probability level. The 0.05 probability level is used extensively in statistical analysis. However, if we wish to impose a higher standard of statistical significance on ourselves, we must employ a smaller probability level. For example, we might wish to adopt a 0.01 probability level rather than a 0.05 probability level. In this case, we would not be willing to reject the null hypothesis unless we obtained results that could be attributed to sampling error no more than 1 out of every 100 samples. In terms of the standard normal distribution, the 0.01 probability level requires us to obtain a z statistic that is smaller than −2.58 or larger than +2.58 in order to reject the null hypothesis of no difference in the average incomes of the minority group and the population as a whole. This implies that the sample mean would have to be much smaller or much larger than the population mean in order to be statistically significant at the 0.01 probability level.

Finally, it must be noted that we have employed what is known in statistics as a two-tailed test because we were prepared to reject the null hypothesis if the z statistic was very large or if the z statistic was very small. However, it is possible to construct a one-tailed test which does not permit us to reject the null hypothesis no matter how large or small the z statistic is unless it is in the predicted direction. The advantage of a one-tailed statistical test is that it enables us to reject the null hypothesis using a less extreme value of the z statistic as long as it is in the predicted direction. For example, we might have a theory that predicts that the average family income of our minority group is less than the average family income of the population as a whole. In this situation, our null hypothesis is that the sample mean is equal to or greater than the population mean. Consequently, we will not reject this null hypothesis unless the sample mean is significantly less than the population mean. Moreover, we will fail to reject this null hypothesis even if the sample mean is much larger than the population mean. Using such a one-tailed statistical test in this example, the sample mean does not have to be much smaller than the population mean in order to be statistically significant. We shall not discuss the use of one-tailed tests in any detail because they are not widely used in regression analysis. In any case, the use of a one-tailed test presupposes that we have a very strong theory that makes an unequivocal assertion about the direction of the relationship between two variables.

CHAPTER 13

Testing Hypotheses
Using the t Test

There is one major problem with using the z test and the normal distribution to test even simple hypotheses. This problem arises, in the case of the test for the significance of a single mean, because we must assume that we know the standard deviation of the variable in the population. Specifically, we must know the population standard deviation in order to estimate the standard error of the sample mean. In practice, of course, we rarely know the values of any of the population parameters. We only know the values of the sample statistics. For many years, statisticians were content to estimate the population standard deviation of a variable using the sample standard deviation of that variable. However, they later discovered that this practice often led to incorrect inferences.

The first difficulty that arises from this approach is that the sample standard deviation of a variable does not provide an accurate estimate of its population standard deviation. Indeed, the sample variance of a variable is a biased estimator of the variance of that variable in the population. *A sample statistic is a biased estimator of a population parameter whenever the average value of this statistic in repeated samples is not equal to the population parameter.* It can be demonstrated that the sample variance systematically underestimates the population variance. Consequently, the z statistic based on the sample standard deviation is inflated to some extent. Fortunately, we can obtain an unbiased estimate of the population variance from the sample variance by adjusting for the number of degrees of freedom lost computing the mean as follows:

$$\hat{\sigma}_x^2 = \frac{N}{N-1} s_x^2$$

The degrees of freedom of a test statistic are determined by sample size and the number of restrictions imposed on these observations in computing the test statistic. For example, in computing the variance of any variable, we lose one degree of freedom because the equation for the variance requires prior knowledge of the mean of that variable. Consequently, in a sample of N observations, N − 1 of the observations are free to assume any value. However, the value of the last observation is fixed by the value of the mean. Specifically, the sum of all the observations must, by definition, equal the number of observations times the mean of these observations. Moreover, as the ratio of the sample size to the number of degrees of freedom in this equation suggests, the bias introduced by using the sample variance to estimate the population variance is relatively small in large samples.

Given this unbiased estimate of the population variance, we can derive the standard error of the sample mean by substituting the standard deviation of the sample for the standard deviation of the population as follows:

$$\hat{\sigma}_{\bar{x}} = \frac{\hat{\sigma}_x}{\sqrt{N}} = \sqrt{\frac{\hat{\sigma}_x^2}{N}} = \sqrt{\left(\frac{N}{N-1}\right)\frac{s_x^2}{N}}$$

$$= \sqrt{\frac{s_x^2}{N-1}} = \frac{s_x}{\sqrt{N-1}}$$

Although this equation provides us with an unbiased estimate of the standard error of the mean, the use of this quantity in the z test statistic will still yield incorrect inferences in small samples. This problem arises because the denominator in the z test statistic is estimated using a sample statistic. In the original z test statistic, the only quantity that varied across samples was the sample mean in the numerator of the test statistic. The population standard deviation in the denominator of this test statistic did not vary across samples, as long as the samples were of the same size. However, whenever the standard error of the mean is estimated using the sample standard deviation, we must contend with the fact that this estimated standard error will also vary across samples. In other words, this z test statistic employs sample statistics that vary from one sample to the next in both the numerator and the denominator. A test statistic comprising the ratio of two sample statistics will not necessarily have a normal distribution.

This problem was eventually solved with the development of the t distribution. The t distribution is the exact sampling distribution associated with a test statistic that employs a sample statistic in the numerator and the standard error of that statistic, estimated from the sample standard deviation, in the denominator. The equation for the t test for the significance of a mean is given as follows:

$$t = \frac{\overline{x} - \mu_x}{\hat{\sigma}_{\overline{x}}} = \frac{\overline{x}}{\hat{\sigma}_{\overline{x}}}$$

where it is assumed that the population mean, μ_x, is equal to zero and where the estimated population standard deviation of the mean is given by:

$$\hat{\sigma}_{\overline{x}} = \frac{s_{\overline{x}}}{\sqrt{N-1}}$$

The t test looks identical to the z test. The only difference is that the t test is based on an estimated population standard deviation, derived from the sample standard deviation, rather than the population standard deviation. Moreover, the statistical significance of this t test is evaluated by referring to critical values associated with the cumulative probability density function of the t distribution. A graph of a t distribution, showing the critical regions for the 0.05 probability level, is presented in Figure 13.1.

It must be noted that the t distribution is actually an entire family of distributions rather than a single distribution. The exact shape of any given t distribution is determined by the number of degrees of freedom associated with the test statistic. For example, the t distribution presented in Figure 13.1 is the distribution of t with 20 degrees of freedom. In the case of the test for the significance of a single mean, the degrees of freedom associated with the t test are equal to N − 1, where N is the sample size. As indicated earlier, one degree of freedom is lost in using the sample mean to compute the standard error of the mean. In general, the t distribution is shorter and fatter than the normal distribution. This implies that the critical regions in the t dis-

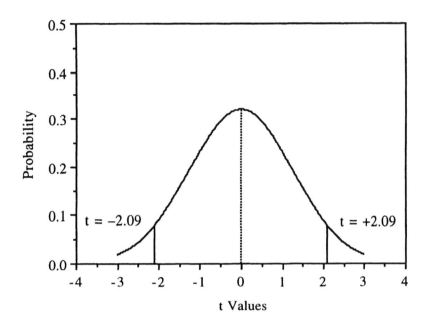

Figure 13.1. t Distribution and Critical t Values

tribution are farther from the mean of the distribution than they are in the normal distribution. In other words, the t test values required to reject the null hypothesis at any given probability level will generally be larger than the corresponding z test values. For example, in the t distribution with 20 degrees of freedom, 95 percent of the cases fall within 2.06 standard errors of the mean. In the normal distribution, it will be recalled, 95 percent of the cases fall within 1.96 standard errors of the mean. Consequently, the t distribution and the normal distribution can provide different results, especially in small samples. However, as sample size becomes extremely large, the t distribution approximates a normal distribution.

Given that there are any number of t distributions, we must refer to a table of critical values for these t distributions in order to assess the statistical significance of any given t test. We begin by determining the number of degrees of freedom associated with our test statistic. In the case of the mean, the number of degrees of freedom will depend entirely on the size of the sample. Next, we choose a particular significance level, such as the 0.05 probability level, and refer to the table of critical values for the appropriate t distribution in order to determine the critical value required to reject the null hypothesis. Finally, we compare our t test value with the appropriate critical value. If our t test value is equal to or larger than this critical value, we must reject the null hypothesis and infer that the difference between the sample mean and the population mean is statistically significant. If our t test value is smaller than the critical value, we must fail to reject the null hypothesis and infer that the difference between the sample mean and the population mean is not statistically significant.

The critical values for the t distribution are given in Table 1 of the statistical tables in the Appendix E. The different probability levels associated with each critical region are given in the columns and the number of degrees of freedom associated with each critical region are given in the rows. An examination of this table reveals that the critical value for t increases as the level of significance becomes more stringent. This implies that the critical region for testing the null hypothesis at the 0.01 probability level is farther from the mean of the sampling distribution, which is equal to zero, than the critical region for testing the null hypothesis at the 0.05 probability level. For example, with 60 degrees of freedom, a t value must be greater than 2.00 in order to be significant at the 0.05 probability level, whereas it must be greater than 2.66 in order to be significant at the 0.01 probability level. An examination of this table also reveals that the critical value for t decreases as the number of degrees of freedom increases. For example, a t value of 2.00 is not significant at the 0.05 probability level with only 40 degrees of freedom but is significant at this same probability level with 120 degrees of freedom. This suggests that the t distribution becomes taller and narrower with larger numbers of degrees of freedom. Indeed, as indicated earlier, the t distribution approximates a normal distribution as the number of degrees of freedom approaches infinity. Consequently, the critical values for the t distribution with an infinite number of degrees of freedom are equal to the corresponding critical values for the z distribution.

CHAPTER 14

The t Test for the Simple Regression Coefficient

Fortunately, it turns out that the t test is applicable to a variety of problems. In particular, it is applicable to the problem of testing the statistical significance of a regression coefficient. Under a set of assumptions that are usually referred to as the Gauss-Markov conditions, the t test can be used to test the significance of a regression coefficient. We will defer a detailed discussion of these assumptions and the consequences of violating them to a later point. For the time being, it is enough to know that these assumptions have to do with the distribution of the errors of prediction. In regression analysis, we are often interested in the simple question of whether or not there is a linear relationship between two variables in the population. Stated in statistical jargon, we wish to test the null hypothesis that the population regression coefficient for the regression of a dependent variable on an independent variable is equal to zero.

The logic of testing the statistical significance of a sample regression coefficient is similar to that we employed in testing the significance of a sample mean. We typically begin with the assumption, stated as the null hypothesis, that the population regression coefficient is equal to zero. However, given our understanding of sampling error, we know that if we draw repeated samples from this population, we will obtain a range of different sample regression coefficients, even if the population regression coefficient is zero. Some of the sample regression coefficients may be equal to zero, but there will also be many positive and many negative regression coefficients as well. Statisticians have proven that the sample least-squares regression coefficient provides an unbiased estimate of the population regression coefficient. In other words, the mean of the sampling distribution of regression coefficients will be equal to the population regression coefficient. Still, any one sample may yield either a positive or a negative regression coefficient as a result of sampling error. Therefore, as we did in the case of the sample mean, we must evaluate a sample regression coefficient in relation to its standard error.

The t test for the significance of a regression coefficient is given by the following equation:

$$t = \frac{b_{yx} - \beta_{yx}}{\hat{\sigma}_b} = \frac{b_{yx}}{s_b}$$

where it is assumed that the population regression coefficient, β_{yx}, is equal to zero. In this case, the t test is simply the ratio of the sample regression coefficient to its standard error. In repeated samples of size N from a population under the null hypothesis, this test statistic follows a t distribution with $N - 2$ degrees of freedom. The degrees of freedom are equal to $N - 2$ in this case because two degrees of freedom are lost in computing the parameters of the simple regression equation: one for the regression coefficient and another for the intercept.

Other things being equal, the value of a t test will be large in absolute terms whenever the value of the sample regression coefficient is large in absolute terms. However, the value of the t test also depends on the magnitude of the standard error of the sample regression coefficient. In short, the deviation of any sample regression coefficient from the population regression coefficient, which is typically assumed to be equal to zero, must be assessed in relation to the standard deviation of the sampling distribution of the regression coefficient. Even if the sample regression coefficient is large, the t test will not be large if the standard error of this coefficient is also large. Indeed, an examination of the t distributions for moderately large samples indicates that a sample regression coefficient must be roughly twice the magnitude of its standard error if it is to be statistically significant at the conventional 0.05 probability level.

There are a number of different equations for the standard error of a simple regression coefficient. The derivation of the standard error of the regression coefficient is somewhat complicated (see Appendix C). We shall restrict our attention to the most interpretable of these given by:

$$s_b = \sqrt{\frac{Var(e)}{Var(x)(N-2)}} = \sqrt{\frac{s_e^2}{s_x^2(N-2)}}$$

This equation demonstrates that the standard error of a regression coefficient depends on the error variance of the regression equation, Var(e), on the size of the sample minus the number of parameters in the simple regression equation, N – 2, and on the variance of the independent variable, Var(x). Moreover, it will be recalled that the error variance can be computed directly from the variance of the dependent variable and the coefficient of determination as follows:

$$Var(e) = Var(y)(1 - r_{yx}^2)$$

In short, the error variance is equal to the variance in the dependent variable that is left unexplained by the independent variable. Therefore, the standard error of the simple regression coefficient can be expressed in terms of four quantities as follows:

$$s_b = \sqrt{\frac{Var(y)(1 - r_{yx}^2)}{Var(x)(N-2)}}$$

It is apparent from this equation that the magnitude of the standard error of a simple regression coefficient is determined by four distinct quantities. The first of these is the variance of the dependent variable, which appears in the numerator of this equation. If the variance of the dependent variable is small, other things being equal, the standard error of the regression coefficient will also be small. The second quantity in the numerator of this equation is equal to one minus the coefficient of determination for the regression equation. If the proportion of the variance in the dependent variable left unexplained by the regression equation is small, other things being equal, the standard error of the regression coefficient will also be small. Another quantity affecting the magnitude of the standard error of the simple regression coefficient is the variance of the independent variable, which appears in the denominator of this equation. If the variance of the independent variable is large, other things being equal, the standard error of the regression coefficient will be small. Finally, the second quantity in the denominator of this equation is sample size minus two. Other things being equal, if the sample size is large, the standard error of the regression coefficient will be small.

We can demonstrate the computation of the t test for the significance of a regression coefficient using the very simple empirical example, presented earlier, of the regression of income on education for four individuals. To begin with, the variances of the observed variables and the coefficient of determination used to compute the error variance are given as follows:

$$Var(e) = Var(y)(1-r_{yx}^2) = s_y^2(1-r_{yx}^2)$$

$$= (51.25)(0.39) = 19.99$$

and

$$Var(x) = 5.0$$

Next, these quantities and the number of degrees of freedom in this simple regression model can be used to obtain the standard error of the regression coefficient as follows:

$$s_b = \sqrt{\frac{Var(e)}{Var(x)(N-2)}} = \sqrt{\frac{19.99}{(5.0)(2)}}$$

$$= \sqrt{\frac{19.99}{10}} = \sqrt{1.999} = 1.414$$

Finally, we can compute the t test for the significance of the regression coefficient by dividing the regression coefficient by its standard error as follows:

$$t = \frac{b_{yx}}{s_b} = \frac{2.5}{1.414} = 1.768$$

In this particular example, the regression coefficient is only 1.7 times larger than its standard error. By consulting a table of critical values for the t distribution with two degrees of freedom, we find that we would require a t test value of at least 4.303 to be significant at the 0.05 significance level. Therefore, this regression coefficient is not statistically significant using the conventional 0.05 significance level. In this case, the lack of statistical significance is almost certainly attributable to the extremely small sample size employed in this example. In small samples, a large t test value is required to achieve significant results because the critical regions are farther from the mean of the sampling distribution. Conversely, in t distributions with 60 or more degrees of freedom, any t test with an absolute value of 2.00 or more is significant at the 0.05 probability level.

Finally, it might be noted that with the advent of computers and calculators, the need for tables of critical values of various distributions, such as the t distribution, has been all but eliminated. Indeed, using a calculator with a cumulative probability density function for the t distribution, it is possible to compute the exact probability that a given regression coefficient could be obtained by chance as a result of sampling error. Specifically, the exact probability of obtaining a regression coefficient as large as 1.738 in a sample of this size by chance is 0.219. In other words, under the null hypothesis that the population regression coefficient is equal to zero, we could have obtained a regression coefficient this large by chance in almost 22 out of every 100 samples of this size.

CHAPTER 15

More Matrix Algebra:
Manipulating Matrices

The simple regression model can be expressed using vector algebra. However, in order to understand fully the multiple regression model, it is necessary to employ matrix algebra. Indeed, a basic familiarity with matrix algebra is also essential to understanding most of the techniques of multivariate statistical analysis. Matrices are simply rectangular arrays of elements. Consider, for example, the matrix G as follows:

$$G = \begin{bmatrix} g_{11} & g_{12} & g_{13} \\ g_{21} & g_{22} & g_{23} \end{bmatrix}$$

This matrix is said to be "2 by 3" because it comprises two rows and three columns (i.e., 2 x 3). Each of the elements in this matrix, g_{ij}, has two subscripts. The first subscript refers to the row of the matrix in which an element appears and the second subscript refers to the column of the matrix in which it appears. For example, the element g_{23} is in the second row and third column of this matrix.

Matrix addition and subtraction are essentially identical to vector addition and subtraction. Two matrices are conformable for either addition or subtraction only if they have the same number of rows and the same number of columns. The elements in the matrix produced by the addition of two matrices are equal to the sum of the elements in the corresponding rows and columns of these two matrices. For example, consider two matrices, H and K, such that:

$$H = \begin{bmatrix} h_{11} & h_{12} \\ h_{21} & h_{22} \\ h_{31} & h_{32} \end{bmatrix} \quad \text{and} \quad K = \begin{bmatrix} k_{11} & k_{12} \\ k_{21} & k_{22} \\ k_{31} & k_{32} \end{bmatrix}$$

The addition of these two matrices is given by:

$$H + K = \begin{bmatrix} h_{11} + k_{11} & h_{12} + k_{12} \\ h_{21} + k_{21} & h_{22} + k_{22} \\ h_{31} + k_{31} & h_{32} + k_{32} \end{bmatrix}$$

Of course, matrix subtraction is performed in a manner analogous to matrix addition.

It is worth noting that a matrix can be seen as the concatenation of two or more vectors. For example, the matrix C, which has two rows and three columns, can be represented as the concatenation of two column vectors, each with three elements, as follows:

$$C = \begin{bmatrix} c_{11} & c_{12} \\ c_{21} & c_{22} \\ c_{31} & c_{32} \end{bmatrix} = \begin{bmatrix} c_1 & c_2 \end{bmatrix}$$

where:

$$c_1 = \begin{bmatrix} c_{11} \\ c_{21} \\ c_{31} \end{bmatrix} \quad \text{and} \quad c_2 = \begin{bmatrix} c_{12} \\ c_{22} \\ c_{32} \end{bmatrix}$$

Alternatively, a matrix can be represented as the concatenation of row vectors as follows:

$$D = \begin{bmatrix} d_{11} & d_{12} & d_{13} \\ \hline d_{21} & d_{22} & d_{23} \end{bmatrix} = \begin{bmatrix} d_1' \\ d_2' \end{bmatrix}$$

where:

$$\mathbf{d}_1' = \begin{bmatrix} d_{11} & d_{12} & d_{13} \end{bmatrix} \quad \text{and} \quad \mathbf{d}_2' = \begin{bmatrix} d_{21} & d_{22} & d_{23} \end{bmatrix}$$

The representation of matrices as concatenations of either row vectors or column vectors is useful because it provides us with a simple method of defining the multiplication of two matrices. According to the rules of matrix algebra, two matrices are conformable for multiplication only if the number of columns in the first or premultiplying matrix is equal to the number of rows in the second or postmultiplying matrix. If two matrices are conformable for multiplication, each element of the product matrix is equal to the scalar product of the corresponding row vector of the premultiplying matrix and the corresponding column vector of the postmultiplying matrix. Therefore, the product of premultiplying matrix $\mathbf{C}$ by matrix $\mathbf{D}$ is given by:

$$\mathbf{D}\mathbf{C} = \begin{bmatrix} \mathbf{d}_1'\mathbf{c}_1 & \mathbf{d}_1'\mathbf{c}_2 & \mathbf{d}_1'\mathbf{c}_3 \\ \mathbf{d}_2'\mathbf{c}_1 & \mathbf{d}_2'\mathbf{c}_2 & \mathbf{d}_2'\mathbf{c}_3 \end{bmatrix}$$

As this example demonstrates, the product matrix has the same number of rows as the premultiplying matrix and the same number of columns as the postmultiplying matrix.

Each element of this product matrix is the scalar product of a specific row vector in the premultiplying matrix and a specific column vector in the postmultiplying matrix. For example, the element in the first row and second column of the product matrix is equal to the scalar product of the vector in the first row of matrix $\mathbf{D}$ and the vector in the second column of matrix $\mathbf{C}$ such that:

$$\mathbf{d}_1'\mathbf{c}_2 = d_{11}c_{12} + d_{12}c_{22} + d_{13}c_{32}$$

The representation of matrix multiplication in terms of the multiplication of row and column vectors also demonstrates the necessity of the conformability condition for matrix multiplication. If each element of the product matrix is the scalar product of a row vector in the premultiplying matrix and a column vector in the postmultiplying matrix, then these vectors must have the same number of elements. Consequently, the number of columns in the first or premultiplying matrix must be equal to the number of rows in the second or postmultiplying matrix. Similarly, the product matrix must necessarily have the same number of rows as the premultiplying matrix and the same number of columns as the postmultiplying matrix.

It is possible, of course, to transpose a matrix, just as it is possible to transpose a vector. Whenever we transpose a matrix, we transpose every column vector in the original matrix into a row vector in the transposed matrix. For example, suppose that we are given the matrix **F** such that:

$$\mathbf{F} = \begin{bmatrix} \mathbf{f_1} & \mathbf{f_2} & \mathbf{f_3} \end{bmatrix} = \begin{bmatrix} f_{11} & f_{12} & f_{13} \\ f_{21} & f_{22} & f_{23} \\ f_{31} & f_{32} & f_{33} \\ f_{41} & f_{42} & f_{43} \end{bmatrix}$$

The transpose of this matrix **F′** is given by:

$$\mathbf{F'} = \begin{bmatrix} \mathbf{f'_1} \\ \mathbf{f'_2} \\ \mathbf{f'_3} \end{bmatrix} = \begin{bmatrix} f_{11} & f_{21} & f_{31} & f_{41} \\ f_{12} & f_{22} & f_{32} & f_{42} \\ f_{13} & f_{23} & f_{33} & f_{43} \end{bmatrix}$$

Moreover, some square matrices are symmetric inasmuch as each element below the main diagonal is equal to the corresponding element above the main diagonal. If a matrix is symmetric, it is equal to its transpose such that:

$$\mathbf{M} = \mathbf{M'}$$

In short, the elements in each row of a symmetric matrix are equal to the elements in the corresponding column of this matrix such that:

$$m_{ij} = m_{ji}$$

Finally, it must noted that, although it is possible to multiply two matrices, it is not possible to divide two matrices. The only operation in matrix algebra that is analogous to division involves the inverse of matrix. Only symmetric matrices have inverses. Most of the symmetric matrices used in regression analysis have inverses. The inverse of any symmetric matrix is defined mathematically as follows:

$$M^{-1}M = MM^{-1} = I$$

where:

$$M = \begin{bmatrix} m_{11} & m_{12} & m_{13} \\ m_{12} & m_{22} & m_{23} \\ m_{13} & m_{23} & m_{33} \end{bmatrix} \quad \text{and} \quad I = \begin{bmatrix} 1 & 0 & 0 \\ 0 & 1 & 0 \\ 0 & 0 & 1 \end{bmatrix}$$

The matrix I is known as an identity matrix. Identity matrices have ones for their main diagonal elements and zeros elsewhere.

Multiplying a matrix by the inverse of another matrix is analogous to dividing the first matrix by the second matrix. These operations are analogous because the result of dividing a number by itself it one, whereas the result of multiplying a matrix by its inverse is an identity matrix with ones in the main diagonal and zeros elsewhere. The inverse of a matrix is very useful in solving systems of equations, especially the normal equations associated with the least-squares estimates of the multiple regression model. Specifically, in order to calculate the least-squares estimates of the parameters of the multiple regression model, we must calculate the inverse of the matrix of covariances among the independent variables. Moreover, the computations required to obtain the inverse of such a matrix are so laborious that they are normally performed by computers. Finally, it must be noted that there are matrices that do not have inverses. *Any matrix that does not have an inverse is known as a singular matrix.* If a matrix of the covariances among the independent variables is singular, it becomes impossible to solve the normal equations for the least-squares estimates of the multiple regression model. Fortunately, the matrices of covariances among the independent variables of a multiple regression model are rarely singular.

CHAPTER 16

The Multiple Regression Model

Simple regression analysis is a very useful statistical technique for examining the relationship between two variables. However, it is not nearly as useful, or powerful, as multiple regression analysis. *Multiple regression employs a linear function of two or more independent variables to explain the variation in a dependent variable.* As such, multiple regression is merely an extension of simple regression. Indeed, the logic of multiple regression analysis is essentially identical to that of simple regression analysis. In simple regression analysis, we predict the observed values of the dependent variable using a linear function of the observed values of the independent variable. Similarly, in multiple regression analysis, we predict the observed values of the dependent variable using a linear function of the observed values of two or more independent variables. We shall begin our discussion of multiple regression using a relatively simple model with only two independent variables such that:

$$y_i = a + b_{y1.2}\, x_1 + b_{y2.1}\, x_2 + e_i$$

where y is the dependent variable, x_1 is the first independent variable, x_2 is the second independent variable, and e is the error of prediction.

Of course, it is possible to express this same equation in terms of vectors such that:

$$y = ua + x_1 b_1 + x_2 b_2 + e$$

where the observations on each variable are given as column vectors as follows:

$$\mathbf{y} = \begin{bmatrix} y_1 \\ y_2 \\ \vdots \\ y_n \end{bmatrix} \qquad \mathbf{x_1} = \begin{bmatrix} x_{11} \\ x_{12} \\ \vdots \\ x_{1n} \end{bmatrix} \qquad \text{and} \qquad \mathbf{x_2} = \begin{bmatrix} x_{21} \\ x_{22} \\ \vdots \\ x_{2n} \end{bmatrix}$$

In this case, the observed x values now have two subscripts: the first refers to the number of the independent variable and the second refers to the number of the observation, such that x_{13} refers to the third observation on variable x_1.

It is important to note that the two vectors of observations on the independent variables can be represented by a single matrix. This matrix of observations on the independent variables can be thought of as the concatenation of the two column vectors of observations on each variable as follows:

$$\mathbf{X} = \begin{bmatrix} \mathbf{x_1} \vdots \mathbf{x_2} \end{bmatrix} = \begin{bmatrix} x_{11} & \vdots & x_{21} \\ x_{12} & \vdots & x_{22} \\ \vdots & & \vdots \\ x_{1n} & \vdots & x_{2n} \end{bmatrix}$$

Similarly, the two partial regression coefficients can be replaced by a vector of partial regression coefficients as follows:

$$\mathbf{b} = \begin{bmatrix} b_{y1.2} \\ b_{y2.1} \end{bmatrix}$$

Therefore, the multiple regression model can be expressed concisely in matrix algebra terms as follows:

$$\mathbf{y} = \mathbf{u}a + \mathbf{Xb} + \mathbf{e}$$

such that:

$$
\begin{bmatrix} y_1 \\ y_2 \\ \vdots \\ y_n \end{bmatrix} = \begin{bmatrix} a \\ a \\ \vdots \\ a \end{bmatrix} + \begin{bmatrix} b_{y1.2}\,x_{11} + b_{y2.1}\,x_{21} \\ b_{y1.2}\,x_{12} + b_{y2.1}\,x_{22} \\ \vdots \qquad \vdots \\ b_{y1.2}\,x_{1n} + b_{y2.1}\,x_{2n} \end{bmatrix} + \begin{bmatrix} e_1 \\ e_2 \\ \vdots \\ e_n \end{bmatrix}
$$

As these equations suggest, the notation used in multiple regression analysis differs slightly from that in simple regression analysis. In particular, the subscripts for the regression coefficients are different. Different notation is required because the regression coefficients used in multiple regression analysis are partial regression coefficients. *A partial regression coefficient represents the expected change in the dependent variable associated with a one unit change in the independent variable, controlling for any changes in the other independent variables.* Consequently, the partial coefficient, $b_{y1.2}$, represents the change in y produced by a one unit change in x_1 holding x_2 constant.

As in the case of simple regression, it is possible to obtain least-squares estimates of the parameters of the multiple regression equation. Specifically, we can obtain least-squares estimates of the partial regression coefficients that will minimize the sum of the squared errors of prediction. These errors of prediction are obtained in the usual manner, as the difference between the observed value and the predicted value on the dependent variable, such that:

$$
\hat{y}_i = a + b_{y1.2}\,x_{1i} + b_{y2.1}\,x_{2i}
$$

and

$$
e_i = y_i - \hat{y}_i
$$

Alternatively, these equations can be expressed in matrix algebra notation as follows:

$$
\hat{\mathbf{y}} = \mathbf{u}a + \mathbf{X}\mathbf{b}
$$

and

$$
\mathbf{e} = \mathbf{y} - \hat{\mathbf{y}}
$$

Table 16.1. Data on Public Expenditures, Economic Openness, and Labor Organization in Seven Major Industrial Nations

Nation	Public expenditures (y)	Economic openness (x_1)	Labor organization (x_2)
Great Britain	47.1	26.8	45.0
Canada	40.5	27.4	27.0
France	48.7	22.6	24.0
West Germany	49.4	28.9	32.0
Italy	50.4	23.0	41.0
Japan	34.0	14.8	16.0
United States	35.2	9.7	21.0

The utility of the multiple regression model can be demonstrated with a relatively simple empirical example. Political scientists have sought to identify the factors that determine the level of public expenditures in modern industrial nations, measured in terms of government spending as a percentage of gross national product. One factor affecting the level of public expenditures is economic openness, measured in terms of exports and imports as a percentage of gross national product. Another factor affecting the level of public expenditures is labor organization, measured in terms of union membership as a percentage of the labor force. Let us assume that we wish to assess the effects of both economic openness and labor organization on the level of public expenditures in seven major industrial nations. The data on these three variables for these seven nations are given in Table 16.1.

The least-squares estimates of the multiple regression equation for the regression of public expenditures on economic openness and labor organization are given as follows:

$$y = u\,(25.05) + x_1\,(0.452) + x_2\,(0.295) + e$$

The computations required to obtain these least-squares estimates of the parameters of this multiple regression equation are laborious. For that reason, we shall postpone a discussion of these computations for the moment. Fortunately, the parameters of this multiple regression model can be interpreted much in the same way as the coefficients of the simple regression model. The intercept can be interpreted as the expected level of public expenditures in a nation in which there was no economic openness and no labor organization. For example, we expect nations without any economic openness or labor organization to devote 25 percent of their Gross National Product to public expenditures. The regression coefficient for variable x_1 can be interpreted as the expected change in the level of public expenditures associated with a one unit change in economic openness, holding labor organization constant. For example, we expect the percent of the Gross National Product devoted to public expenditures to increase by 0.45 percent for every 1 percent increase in economic openness, holding labor organization constant. Conversely, the regression coefficient for variable x_2 can be interpreted as the expected change in the level of public expenditures associated with a one unit change in labor organization, holding economic openness constant.

CHAPTER 17

Normal Equations and
Partial Regression Coefficients

It can be demonstrated, using calculus, that the ordinary least-squares estimates of the partial regression coefficients for a multiple regression equation are given by a series of equations known as the *normal equations*. A derivation of the normal equations is presented in Appendix D. The simplest form for these equations is in terms of the correlations among the variables. In short, we can assume, without any loss of generality, that all of the variables are in standard form. Specifically, the normal equations can be written such that the correlation between the dependent variable and each independent variable can be expressed as a linear function of the standardized partial regression coefficients and the correlations among the independent variables. For example, the normal equations for a multiple regression equation with three independent variables can be written as follows:

$$r_{y1} = b^*_{y1.23} + b^*_{y2.13} r_{12} + b^*_{y3.12} r_{13}$$

$$r_{y2} = b^*_{y1.23} r_{21} + b^*_{y2.13} + b^*_{y3.12} r_{23}$$

$$r_{y3} = b^*_{y1.23} r_{31} + b^*_{y2.13} r_{32} + b^*_{y3.12}$$

The correlations between the dependent variable and the independent variable, r_{yi}, and the correlations between the independent variables, r_{ij}, can be readily calculated from the observations on these variables.

However, the standardized partial regression coefficients, $b^*_{yi.jk}$, can only be obtained by solving these equations.

Fortunately, this system of normal equations can be written more concisely in matrix algebra as follows:

$$\mathbf{r}_{yx} = \mathbf{R}_{xx}\, \mathbf{b}^*_{yx}$$

Specifically, the column vector of correlations between the dependent variable and the independent variables, $\mathbf{r}_{yx}$, is equal to the product of the matrix of correlations among the independent variables, $\mathbf{R}_{xx}$, postmultiplied by the column vector of standardized partial regression coefficients, $\mathbf{b}^*_{yx}$. The matrix of correlations among the independent variables is given by:

$$\mathbf{R}_{xx} = \begin{bmatrix} 1 & r_{12} & r_{13} \\ r_{21} & 1 & r_{23} \\ r_{31} & r_{32} & 1 \end{bmatrix}$$

The main diagonal elements of this correlation matrix are set to ones because standardized variables have variances of one. Also, this correlation matrix is symmetric, inasmuch as r_{ij} is equal to r_{ji}, such that:

$$\mathbf{R}_{xx} = \begin{bmatrix} 1 & r_{12} & r_{13} \\ r_{12} & 1 & r_{23} \\ r_{13} & r_{23} & 1 \end{bmatrix}$$

Next, the column vector of correlations between the dependent variable and the independent variables is given by:

$$\mathbf{r}_{yx} = \begin{bmatrix} r_{y1} \\ r_{y2} \\ r_{y3} \end{bmatrix}$$

Finally, the column vector of standardized partial regression coefficients between the dependent variable and the independent variables is given by:

$$\mathbf{b}_{yx}^{*} = \begin{bmatrix} b_{y1.23}^{*} \\ b_{y2.13}^{*} \\ b_{y3.12}^{*} \end{bmatrix}$$

The problem is to solve this system of normal equations for the column vector of unknown regression coefficients, $\mathbf{b}_{yx}^{*}$, given the matrix of observed correlations among the independent variables, $\mathbf{R}_{xx}$, and the column vector of observed correlations between these independent variables and the dependent variable, $\mathbf{r}_{yx}$. As we shall see, the solution to this system of equations requires us to compute the inverse of the matrix of correlations among the independent variables, $\mathbf{R}_{xx}^{-1}$, such that:

$$\mathbf{R}_{xx}^{-1} \mathbf{r}_{yx} = \mathbf{I}$$

It must be noted that some matrices are singular inasmuch as they do not have inverses. In the case of a correlation matrix, this situation can occur only if one of the independent variables is an exact linear function of the other independent variables.

Given the inverse of a correlation matrix, it is not difficult to calculate the standardized partial regression coefficients. First, we premultiply both sides of the normal equations by the inverse of the matrix of correlations between the independent variables, $\mathbf{R}_{xx}^{-1}$, as follows:

$$\mathbf{r}_{yx} = \mathbf{R}_{xx} \mathbf{b}_{yx}^{*}$$

$$\mathbf{R}_{xx}^{-1}(\mathbf{r}_{yx}) = \mathbf{R}_{xx}^{-1}(\mathbf{R}_{xx} \mathbf{b}_{yx}^{*})$$

$$\mathbf{R}_{xx}^{-1} \mathbf{r}_{yx} = \mathbf{R}_{xx}^{-1} \mathbf{R}_{xx} \mathbf{b}_{yx}^{*} = \mathbf{I} \mathbf{b}_{yx}^{*}$$

$$\mathbf{R}_{xx}^{-1} \mathbf{r}_{yx} = \mathbf{b}_{yx}^{*}$$

Therefore, once we have calculated the inverse of the matrix of correlations among the independent variables, $\mathbf{R}_{xx}^{-1}$, we simply postmultiply it by the column vector of correlations between the dependent variable and the independent variables, $\mathbf{r}_{yx}$, in order to obtain the column vector of standardized partial regression coefficients between the dependent variable and the independent variables, b^*_{yx}.

We can demonstrate these computations with a simple example involving three independent variables. We begin by calculating the matrix of correlations among the three independent variables such that:

$$\mathbf{R_{xx}} = \begin{bmatrix} 1.00 & 0.35 & 0.24 \\ 0.35 & 1.00 & 0.38 \\ 0.24 & 0.38 & 1.00 \end{bmatrix}$$

We also calculate the column vector of correlations between the dependent variable and the three independent variables such that:

$$\mathbf{r_{yx}} = \begin{bmatrix} 0.54 \\ 0.78 \\ 0.35 \end{bmatrix}$$

Next, we calculate the inverse of the matrix of correlations among the independent variables. Specifically, the inverse of this particular correlation matrix is given by:

$$\mathbf{R^{-1}_{xx}} = \begin{bmatrix} 1.15 & -0.34 & -0.15 \\ -0.34 & 1.27 & -0.39 \\ -0.15 & -0.39 & 1.18 \end{bmatrix}$$

We can verify that this matrix is, indeed, the inverse of the matrix of correlations among the independent variables as follows:

$$\mathbf{R^{-1}_{xx} R_{xx}} = \mathbf{I} = \begin{bmatrix} 1.00 & 0.00 & 0.00 \\ 0.00 & 1.00 & 0.00 \\ 0.00 & 0.00 & 1.00 \end{bmatrix}$$

Finally, in order to calculate the column vector of standardized partial regression coefficients, it is necessary to premultiply the column vector of correlations between the dependent variable and the independent variables by the inverse of the matrix of correlations among the independent variables as follows:

$$b_{yx}^* = R_{xx}^{-1} r_{yx} = \begin{bmatrix} 0.30 \\ 0.67 \\ 0.02 \end{bmatrix}$$

It must be noted that these are *standardized* partial regression coefficients. We can obtain the corresponding unstandardized partial regression coefficients simply by multiplying each standardized partial regression coefficients by the ratio of the standard deviation of the dependent variable to the standard deviation of the independent variable. For example, a given unstandardized partial regression coefficient, $b_{yi.jk}$, can be obtained from its corresponding standardized partial regression coefficient, $b_{yi.jk}^*$, as follows:

$$b_{yi.jk} = b_{yi.jk}^* \left(\frac{s_y}{s_i} \right)$$

where s_y is the standard deviation of the dependent variable and s_i is the standard deviation of independent variable x_i. Similarly, given the unstandardized partial regression coefficients and the means of both the dependent and independent variables, it is possible to compute the intercept for the multiple regression equation with unstandardized variables as follows:

$$a = \bar{y} - b_{y1.23}\bar{x}_1 - b_{y2.13}\bar{x}_2 - b_{y3.12}\bar{x}_3$$

In short, there are exact mathematical correspondences between the parameters of a multiple regression model obtained using standardized variables and the parameters of the same model obtained using unstandardized variables.

CHAPTER 18

Partial Regression and
Residualized Variables

Partial regression coefficients are the most important parameters of the multiple regression model. They measure the expected change in the dependent variable associated with a one unit change in an independent variable holding the other independent variables constant. This interpretation of partial regression coefficients is very important because independent variables are often correlated with one another. Unfortunately, the concept of partial regression can be somewhat difficult to understand because it relies upon the notion of statistical control. However, this difficulty can be alleviated somewhat if we view a partial regression coefficient as equivalent to a simple regression coefficient involving an independent variable that has had the effects of the other independent variables removed from it.

In order to understand the logic of partial regression coefficients more clearly, let us consider the case of a multiple regression equation with two independent variables. In this case, the partial regression coefficient for the effect of the first independent variable, x_1, on the dependent variable, y, controlling for the effect of the second independent variable, x_2, is given by:

$$b_{y1.2} = \frac{\text{Cov}(y, x_{1.2})}{\text{Var}(x_{1.2})}$$

This equation for the partial regression coefficient is merely an extension of the more familiar equation for the simple regression coefficient. The only difference is that this equation involves an independent variable, $x_{1.2}$, that is a residualized variable. Specifically, this residualized variable is that component of the first independent variable, x_1, that cannot be explained or predicted by the second independent variable, x_2.

Fortunately, residualized variables are relatively easy to compute. In this case, we begin by estimating the parameters of the auxiliary regression equation for the regression of the first independent variable, x_1, on the second independent variable, x_2, as follows:

$$x_1 = ua + x_2 b_{12} + e$$

Next, we use the intercept and the regression coefficient from this auxiliary regression equation to compute the predicted values of the first independent variable, $\hat{x}_1$, as follows:

$$\hat{x}_1 = ua + x_2 b_{12}$$

Finally, we subtract these predicted values from the observed values on the first independent variable to obtain the values of the associated residualized variable, $x_{1.2}$, as follows:

$$x_{1.2} = x_1 - \hat{x}_1$$

This residualized variable, $x_{1.2}$, represents that component or part of the first independent variable, x_1, that cannot be explained or predicted by the second independent variable, x_2.

It might be noted that we can employ the same procedure in order to obtain the partial regression coefficient for the regression of the dependent variable, y, on the second independent variable, x_2, controlling for the first independent variable, x_1. Specifically this partial regression coefficient is given by:

$$b_{y2.1} = \frac{Cov(y, x_{2.1})}{Var(x_{2.1})}$$

where $x_{2.1}$ is the residualized variable obtained from the auxiliary regression of the second independent variable, x_2, on the first independent variable, x_1.

We can illustrate this interpretation of the partial regression coefficient using the regression of economic openness, x_1, on public expenditures, y, controlling for labor organization, x_2, among seven major industrial nations. We begin by regressing economic openness, x_1, on labor organization, x_2, as follows:

$$x_1 = u (9.23) + x_2 (0.430) + e$$

Next, we compute the predicted values of economic openness, $\hat{x}_1$, using the parameters of this equation as follows:

$$\hat{x}_1 = u (9.23) + x_2 (0.430)$$

Finally, we compute the residualized values of economic openness with respect to labor organization, $x_{1.2}$, by subtracting the predicted values, $\hat{x}_1$, from the observed values, x_1, as follows:

$$x_{1.2} = x_1 - \hat{x}_1$$

The observed values, predicted values, and residualized values obtained from the auxiliary regression of economic openness on labor organization for seven major industrial nations are given in Table 18.1.

Given these residualized values of economic openness, it is possible to compute the partial regression coefficient between public expenditures and economic openness residualized with respect to labor organization as follows:

$$\text{Var}(x_{1.2}) = 25.761$$

$$\text{Cov}(y, x_{1.2}) = 11.631$$

$$b_{y1.2} = \frac{\text{Cov}(y, x_{1.2})}{\text{Var}(x_{1.2})} = \frac{11.631}{25.761} = 0.452$$

This simple regression coefficient is equal to the partial regression coefficient for this variable in the multiple regression equation presented earlier.

Table 18.1. Observed Values, Predicted Values, and Residualized
Values from the Regression of Economic Openness
on Labor Organization

Nation	Observed values (x_1)	Predicted values $(\hat{x}_1)$	Residual values $(x_{1.2})$
Great Britain	26.8	28.6	-1.8
Canada	27.4	20.8	6.6
France	22.6	19.5	3.1
West Germany	28.9	23.0	5.9
Italy	23.0	26.9	-3.9
Japan	14.8	16.1	-1.3
United States	9.7	18.3	-8.6

This procedure for obtaining the partial regression coefficient in
the case of two independent variables can be extended to higher-order
partial regression coefficients for multiple regression equations in
which there are more than two independent variables. For example,
the partial regression coefficient for the regression of a dependent
variable, x_1, on a given independent variable, y, controlling for two
other independent variables, x_2 and x_3, is given by:

$$b_{y1.23} = \frac{Cov(y, x_{1.23})}{Var(x_{1.23})}$$

In this case, the first independent variable, x_1, has been residualized
with respect to both the second and third independent variables, x_2
and x_3. This residualized variable can be computed from the auxiliary regression equation for the regression of the first independent
variable, x_1, on the second and third independent variables, x_2 and x_3,
as follows:

$$x_1 = ua + x_2 b_{12.3} + x_3 b_{13.2} + e$$

$$\hat{x}_1 = ua + x_2 b_{12.3} + x_3 b_{13.2}$$

$$x_{1.23} = x_1 - \hat{x}_1$$

This approach to computing partial regression coefficients can be extended to include any number of independent variables.

This interpretation of the partial regression coefficient leads to another important conclusion. Specifically, it can be demonstrated that the partial regression coefficient for an independent variable that is uncorrelated with the other independent variables in a multiple regression equation is equal to its simple regression coefficient in a simple regression equation predicting the same dependent variable. This situation obtains because the residualized independent variable, in this case, has the same variance and the same covariance with the dependent variable as the unresidualized independent variable. Whenever one independent variable is uncorrelated with the other independent variables, the partial regression coefficients in the auxiliary regression equation between this independent variable and the other independent variables are all equal to zero. Moreover, if these partial regression coefficients are equal to zero, the intercept in this auxiliary regression equation is equal to the mean of the dependent variable in this equation. Consequently, the residualized variable is simply the unresidualized variable expressed in mean deviation form. Of course, a regression coefficient is unaffected by the transformation of variables to mean deviation form.

CHAPTER 19

The Coefficient of Determination in Multiple Regression

In the case of simple regression analysis, the coefficient of determination measures the proportion of the variance in the dependent variable explained by the independent variable. This coefficient is computed using either the variance of the errors of prediction or the variance of the predicted values in relation to the variance of the observed values on the dependent variable as follows:

$$r_{yx}^2 = \left(\frac{\mathrm{Var}(\hat{y})}{\mathrm{Var}(y)} \right) = 1 - \left(\frac{\mathrm{Var}(e)}{\mathrm{Var}(y)} \right)$$

This equation for the coefficient of determination in simple regression analysis can easily be extended to the case of multiple regression analysis. The variances of the predicted values and the errors of prediction in simple regression have direct counterparts in multiple regression. In the case of two independent variables, for example, the following equations obtain:

$$\hat{y} = \mathbf{u}a + x_1 b_{y1.2} + x_2 b_{y2.1}$$

$$e = y - \hat{y}$$

In short, the addition of independent variables to the regression model does not affect the equations for computing either the predicted values or the errors of prediction.

Moreover, the fundamental relationship between the variance of the dependent variable, y, the variance of the predicted values, $\hat{y}$, and the variance of the errors of prediction, e, remains the same, such that:

$$Var(y) = Var(\hat{y}) + Var(e)$$

Therefore, the coefficient of determination in multiple regression analysis has exactly the same definition as it does in simple regression analysis, such that:

$$R^2_{y.12} = \left(\frac{Var(\hat{y})}{Var(y)} \right) = 1 - \left(\frac{Var(e)}{Var(y)} \right)$$

In other words, the interpretation of the coefficient of determination remains the same regardless of how many variables there are in the regression equation.

It will be noticed that the notation used to denote the coefficient of determination is different in the case of multiple regression. The lower case r is replaced with an upper case R and the subscript contains a dot that separates the dependent variable from the independent variables. For example, $R^2_{y.12}$ refers to the proportion of the variance in the dependent variable, y, explained by two independent variables, x_1 and x_2. It will be recalled that the coefficient of determination is an important goodness-of-fit statistic. As such, it measures how well a regression model "fits" the data. It ranges from zero, when there is no relationship between the dependent variable and a linear function of the independent variables, to one, when there is an exact relationship between the dependent variable and a linear function of the independent variables. This goodness-of-fit statistic is very useful because it enables us to compare different regression equations in terms of how well each of them fits the data. Other things being equal, we will normally prefer the regression model with the largest coefficient of determination.

The computations required to obtain the coefficient of determination in a multiple regression model can be demonstrated using the example of the regression of public expenditures, y, on economic openness, x_1, and labor organization, x_2, where the equation for the predicted values of the dependent variable is given by:

$$\hat{y} = u (25.05) + x_1 (0.452) + x_2 (0.295)$$

Table 19.1. Observed Values, Predicted Values, and Errors of Prediction for Dependent Variable in Multiple Regression Model

Nation	Observed value (y)	Predicted value ($\hat{y}$)	Error of prediction (e)
Great Britain	47.1	50.4	-3.3
Canada	40.5	45.4	-4.9
France	48.7	42.4	6.3
West Germany	49.4	47.5	1.9
Italy	50.4	47.5	2.9
Japan	34.0	36.5	-2.5
United States	35.2	35.6	-0.4

Consequently, the errors of prediction associated with this multiple regression equation can be computed as follows:

$$e = y - \hat{y}$$

The observed public expenditure values, the predicted public expenditure values, and the errors of prediction obtained using this multiple regression equation are given in Table 19.1.

In order to compute the coefficient of determination, we must first compute the variance of the dependent variable, y, and the variance of either the predicted values of the dependent variable, $\hat{y}$, or the errors of prediction, e, as follows:

$$\text{Var(y)} = \frac{1}{N}(y'y - \bar{y}'\bar{y}) = \frac{1}{N}\Sigma y_i^2 - \bar{y}^2$$

$$= 1943.70 - 1902.18 = 41.52$$

$$\text{Var}(\hat{y}) = \frac{1}{N}(\hat{y}'\hat{y} - \bar{y}'\bar{y}) = \frac{1}{N}\Sigma\hat{y}_i^2 - \bar{y}^2$$

$$= 1930.36 - 1902.18 = 28.18$$

and

$$\text{Var}(e) = \frac{1}{N}(e'e) = \frac{1}{N}\Sigma e_i^2$$

$$= 13.34$$

Given these quantities, the coefficient of determination for this regression equation can be computed as follows:

$$R_{y.12}^2 = \left(\frac{\text{Var}(\hat{y})}{\text{Var}(y)}\right) = \frac{28.18}{41.52} = 0.679$$

or, alternatively, as follows:

$$R_{y.12}^2 = 1 - \left(\frac{\text{Var}(e)}{\text{Var}(y)}\right) = 1 - \left(\frac{13.36}{41.52}\right)$$

$$= 1 - 0.321 = 0.679$$

This coefficient of determination indicates that economic openness, x_1, and labor organization, x_2, explain 67.9 percent of the variance in public expenditures, y.

It is worth noting that there is a computational equation for the variance of the predicted value of the dependent variable that involves only the partial regression coefficients and the covariances of the independent variables and the dependent variable. Specifically, we can obtain the variance of the predicted value of the dependent variable as follows:

$$\text{Var}(\hat{y}) = b_{y1.2}\,\text{Cov}(y,x_1) + b_{y2.1}\,\text{Cov}(y,x_2)$$

This computational equation for the coefficient of determination can be simplified if we assume that all of the variables are in standard form. This assumption is trivial because the coefficient of determination for a regression equation is not affected by the transformation of the variables to standard form. In such a case, the partial regression coefficients become standardized partial regression coefficients and the covariances of each independent variable with the dependent variable become simple correlations:

$$\text{Var}(\hat{z}_y) \; = \; b^*_{y1.2} \, r_{y1} \; + \; b^*_{y2.1} \, r_{y2}$$

Moreover, under this assumption, the variance of the observed values on the dependent variable is equal to one. Consequently, the coefficient of determination can be expressed as follows:

$$R^2_{y.12} \; = \; \text{Var}(\hat{z}_y) \; = \; b^*_{y1.2} \, r_{y1} \; + \; b^*_{y2.1} \, r_{y2}$$

In other words, the coefficient of determination is equal to the sum of the products of each standardized partial regression coefficient and the corresponding simple correlation coefficient between that independent variable and the dependent variable.

We can demonstrate the use of this computational equation for the coefficient of determination using the empirical example of the multiple regression of public expenditures, y, on economic openness, x_1, and labor organization, x_2, in seven major industrial nations, such that:

$$R^2_{y.12} \; = \; b^*_{y1.2} \, r_{y1} \; + \; b^*_{y2.1} \, r_{y2}$$

$$= \; (0.462)(0.748) \; + \; (0.448)(0.743)$$

$$= \; 0.346 \; + \; 0.333 \; = \; 0.679$$

It might be noted that this computational equation for the coefficient of determination might seem to suggest a procedure for identifying the proportion of the variance in the dependent variable explained by each independent variable. Unfortunately, this decomposition of the coefficient of determination is not especially useful. Indeed, we shall soon examine a much more useful procedure for identifying the proportion of the variance in the dependent variable explained by each independent variable.

CHAPTER 20

Standard Errors of Partial Regression Coefficients

Simple hypothesis testing, involving the statistical significance of a single regression coefficient, is conducted in the same manner in the multiple regression model as it is in the simple regression model. Indeed, the statistical test for the significance of a single partial regression coefficient is merely an extension of that for the simple regression coefficient. Specifically, the t test value for the significance of a partial regression coefficient is obtained by dividing the coefficient by its standard error as follows:

$$ t = \frac{b_{yi.jk}}{s_{b_i}} $$

where $b_{yi.jk}$ is the partial regression coefficient for the regression of the dependent variable y on the independent variable x_i, controlling for the independent variables x_j and x_k, and s_{b_i} is the standard error of this partial regression coefficient.

Although the t tests for simple and partial regression coefficients are identical, the equation for the standard error of a partial regression coefficient is a bit more complicated than the equation for the standard error of a simple regression coefficient. In particular, the equation for the standard error of the partial regression coefficient, $b_{yi.jk}$, is given as follows:

$$s_{b_i} = \sqrt{\frac{Var(e)}{Var(x_i)\,(N-k-1)\,(1-R_{i.jk}^2)}}$$

where $Var(e)$ is the error variance of the multiple regression equation and $Var(x_i)$ is the variance of the independent variable, x_i. These quantities are the same as those used to compute the standard error of the simple regression coefficient. However, this equation contains the quantity $(N - k - 1)$, rather than the quantity $(N - 2)$, in the denominator. This quantity refers to the degrees of freedom associated with this statistic, where N is the number of cases and k is the number of independent variables in the multiple regression equation. Moreover, the quantity $(1-R_{i.jk}^2)$ has been added to the denominator. This quantity is equal to the proportion of the variance in a particular independent variable that is left unexplained by the other independent variables in the regression equation.

It must be noted that the interpretation of this equation can be simplified by the fact that the error variance of a multiple regression equation is equal to the product of the variance of the dependent variable and the proportion of variance in the dependent variable that is not explained by the independent variables such that:

$$Var(e) = Var(y)\,(1-R_{y.ijk}^2)$$

Therefore, the equation for standard error of the partial regression coefficient can be expressed as follows:

$$s_{b_{yi.jk}} = \sqrt{\frac{Var(y)\,(1 - R_{y.ijk}^2)}{Var(x_i)\,(N-k-1)\,(1 - R_{i.jk}^2)}}$$

It is important to note that some of the quantities in this equation vary from one partial regression coefficient to another, whereas other quantities are the same for all of the partial regression coefficients in a given multiple regression equation. Specifically, the two quantities in the numerator of this equation, the variance of the dependent variable and the proportion of the variance in that variable that is not explained by the multiple regression equation, are the same for each partial regression coefficient. Conversely, two of the quantities in the denominator, the variance of each independent variable and the proportion of the variance in that independent variable that is not explained by the other independent variables, are likely to be different for each partial regression coefficient. Of course, the number of degrees of freedom in the denominator is the same for each partial regression coefficient.

This form of the equation identifies all of the factors that determine the magnitude of the standard error of a partial regression coefficient. In order to obtain statistically significant results, the standard error must be small in comparison to the partial regression coefficient. Looking at the numerator of this equation, we see immediately that the standard error will be small if the independent variables in the regression equation explain a relatively large proportion of the variance in the dependent variable and if the variance of the dependent variable is relatively small. Conversely, looking at the denominator of this equation, we see that the standard error will be small if the proportion of the variance in a given independent variable explained by the other independent variables in the regression equation is relatively small, the variance of that independent variable is relatively large, and the number of observations relative to the number of independent variables is large. Consequently, other things being equal, the partial regression coefficient for an independent variable is more likely to be statistically significant whenever that variable is uncorrelated with the other independent variables.

In order to examine how the standard error of an independent variable is affected by its correlation with the other independent variables, let us consider the hypothetical case of a multiple regression equation with three independent variables in which the first independent variable happens to be only minimally related to the other two independent variables. Specifically, we shall assume that the coefficient of determination between the first independent variable, x_1, and the two other independent variables, x_2 and x_3, is only 0.05. In other words, these two independent variables explain only 5 percent of the variance in the first independent variable. Moreover, we shall assume that the coefficient of determination for the overall multiple regression equation is 0.40. In short, the three independent variables explain 40 percent of the variance in the dependent variable. For the sake of convenience, we shall also assume that all of the variables have variances that are equal to 2.0 and that there are 54 cases in our sample. Given these quantities, the standard error of the partial regression coefficient for the first independent variable, x_1, can be computed as follows:

$$s_{b_1} = \sqrt{\frac{\text{Var}(y)\,(1 - R^2_{y.123})}{\text{Var}(x_1)(N - k - 1)(1 - R^2_{1.23})}}$$

$$= \sqrt{\frac{(2.0)\,(0.60)}{(2.0)\,(50)\,(0.95)}}$$

$$= \sqrt{\frac{1.2}{95}} = \sqrt{0.126} = 0.355$$

Next, let us consider the standard error for an independent variable that happens to be highly correlated with the other independent variables in the regression equation. Specifically, we shall assume that the coefficient of determination between the first independent variable and the two other independent variables is 0.80. In other words, these two independent variables, x_2 and x_3, explain 80 percent of the variance in the first independent variable, x_1. Otherwise, we shall assume that the variances of the variables, the number of cases, and the proportion of the variance in the dependent variable explained by the three independent variables remain unchanged. Given these quantities, the standard error of the partial regression coefficient for the first independent variable, x_1, can be computed as follows:

$$s_{b_1} = \sqrt{\frac{(2.0)\,(0.60)}{(2.0)\,(50)\,(0.20)}}$$

$$= \sqrt{\frac{1.2}{20}} = \sqrt{0.600} = 0.770$$

Obviously, the standard error of an independent variable that is highly related to the other independent variables is much larger than the standard error of an independent variable that is not highly related to the other independent variables.

Whenever an independent variable is highly correlated with the other independent variables in a multiple regression equation, we face a serious statistical problem known as multicollinearity. *Multicollinearity is present whenever an independent variable is very highly correlated with the other independent variables in a multiple regression equation.* Multicollinearity is a problem in multiple regression models because the partial regression coefficient for any collinear variable is highly unstable. In other words, the partial regression coefficient for a given variable is likely to vary greatly from one sample to the next due to slight variations in the correlations among the variables across these samples. In fact, we can usually detect the presence of multicollinearity in a multiple regression equation from the magnitudes of the standard errors of the partial regression coefficients. Whenever the standard error of a partial regression coefficient is large in relation to the partial regression coefficient itself, it is likely that the independent variable is highly correlated with the other independent variables. As we shall see later, multicollinearity can be a vexing problem. Two independent variables may each be highly correlated with a particular dependent variable. However, it is difficult to estimate the effect of one independent variable on the dependent variable, holding constant the other independent variable, whenever these two independent variables are highly correlated with one another.

CHAPTER 21

The Incremental Contributions
of Variables

In multiple regression analysis, we often want to know how much of the variance in a dependent variable is explained by one variable or set of variables above and beyond the variance already explained by another variable or set of variables. In short, we want to know the *incremental contribution* of a variable or set of variables in explaining the variance in the dependent variable. Technically, the answer to this question is provided by the *coefficient of semipartial determination*. It is given this name because it is equal to the squared semipartial correlation coefficient. *The coefficient of semipartial determination measures the proportion of the variance in the dependent variable explained by one or more independent variables above and beyond that already explained by one or more other independent variables.*

In order to understand this coefficient, let us consider the case of orthogonal independent variables. *Two or more independent variables are said to be orthogonal whenever they are uncorrelated with one another.* It can be demonstrated that, whenever two independent variables are orthogonal, the coefficient of determination for their multiple regression equation is equal to the sum of the two coefficients of determination for their separate simple regression equations as follows:

$$R^2_{y.12} = b^*_{y1.2}\, r_{y1} + b^*_{y2.1}\, r_{y2}$$

$$= r^2_{y1} + r^2_{y2}$$

We obtain this equation whenever the independent variables are uncorrelated, because each partial regression coefficient is equal to the respective simple regression coefficient, which is equal to the correlation coefficient between the dependent variable and the independent variable. In practice, however, the independent variables in a multiple regression equation are typically correlated with one another to some extent. In these cases, the sum of their separate coefficients of determination will exceed their combined coefficient of determination. This occurs because some of the variance in the dependent variable explained by one independent variable is variance that is already explained by the other correlated independent variable.

Specifically, the coefficient of determination between a dependent variable and two correlated independent variables is equal to the sum of the simple coefficient of determination for the first independent variable and the coefficient of semipartial determination for the second independent variable such that:

$$R^2_{y.12} = r^2_{y1} + R^2_{y(2.1)}$$

In this equation, the first term on the right is the simple coefficient of determination between the dependent variable and the first independent variable. The next term is the coefficient of semipartial determination, representing the incremental contribution of the second variable above and beyond the contribution of the first variable. There are different ways of computing these coefficients of semipartial determination, but the easiest method by far is to calculate the incremental contribution of a variable as follows:

$$R^2_{y(2.1)} = R^2_{y.12} - r^2_{y1}$$

In this instance, we compute the incremental contribution of a variable by simply taking the difference between the proportion of the variance in the dependent variable that is explained by both independent variables and the proportion of the variance that is explained by the first independent variable alone.

It is important to understand that the coefficient of semipartial correlation for a particular independent variable is equal to the coefficient of determination between the dependent variable and an independent variable that has been residualized with respect to the other independent variables. In short, the incremental contribution of a variable is equal to the variance in the dependent variable explained by an independent variable that has had all of the variance explained by the other independent variables removed from it. We can demonstrate this property using a residualized variable obtained from the auxiliary regression of the second independent variable on the first independent variable as follows:

$$x_2 = ua + x_1 b_{21} + e_2$$

$$\hat{x}_2 = ua + x_1 b_{21}$$

$$x_{2.1} = x_2 - \hat{x}_2$$

These equations define a residualized variable, $x_{2.1}$, that represents that component of the second independent variable, x_2, that is not explained by the first independent variable, x_1. As demonstrated earlier, there are three steps involved in calculating this residual variable. First, the second independent variable is regressed on the first independent variable. Next, the intercept and regression coefficient from this equation and the observed values on the first independent variable are used to create predicted values on the second independent variable. Finally, these predicted values are subtracted from the observed values on the second independent variable to create residualized values for the second independent variable with respect to the first independent variable.

It can be demonstrated that the coefficient of determination between this residualized component of the second independent variable and the dependent variable, $r_{y(2.1)}^2$, is equal to the coefficient of semipartial determination between these two variables controlling for the first independent variable, $R_{y.1(2.1)}^2$, such that:

$$r_{y(2.1)}^2 = R_{y.1(2.1)}^2$$

In short, the creation of a residual variable, by removing the effect of the first independent variable from the second independent variable, is equivalent to creating a second independent variable that is orthogonal or uncorrelated with the first independent variable. This result obtains because the errors of prediction in any regression equation are, by definition, uncorrelated with the independent variable in that regression equation. Therefore, one direct interpretation of the coefficient of semipartial determination is that it measures the incremental contribution of a variable in terms of how much of the variance in the dependent variable is explained by that part of the second independent variable that is uncorrelated with the first independent variable.

In order to understand this interpretation of the coefficient of semipartial determination, let us consider the familiar example of the multiple regression of public expenditures on economic openness and labor organization in seven major industrial nations. The coefficient of semipartial determination allows us to examine the proportion of the variance in public expenditures explained by labor organization, over and above that already explained by economic openness. To begin with, we must estimate two separate regression equations and obtain their respective coefficients of determination in order to determine how much of the variance in the dependent variable is explained by each equation. The first equation is the multiple regression equation explaining public expenditures, y, using both economic openness, x_1, and labor organization, x_2, as independent variables. The second equation is a simple regression equation explaining public expenditures, y, using only economic openness, x_1, as a predictor. The results of these analyses and the computation of the coefficient of semipartial determination are given as follows:

$$R^2_{y.12} = 0.679$$

$$r^2_{y1} = 0.560$$

$$R^2_{y(2.1)} = R^2_{y.12} - r^2_{y1} = 0.679 - 0.560 = 0.119$$

Moreover, it can be demonstrated that the same result obtains using the coefficient of determination between public expenditures, y, and the residual variable, $x_{2.1}$, representing that component of economic openness, x_2, that is not explained by labor organization, x_2, as follows:

$$r^2_{y(2.1)} = 0.119$$

These results tell us several things. Altogether, economic openness and labor organization explain 68 percent of the variance in public expenditures. However, economic openness alone explains 56 percent of the variance in public expenditures. Therefore, labor organization explains only 12 percent of the variance in public expenditures not already explained by economic openness.

The decomposition of the coefficient of determination into a series of coefficients of semipartial determination can be extended to any number of variables. This coefficient of semipartial determination can be computed simply as the increment in the coefficient of determination produced by the inclusion of this variable into the regression equation. In the case of three independent variables, for example, the equations are as follows:

$$R^2_{y.123} = r^2_{y1} + R^2_{y(2.1)} + R^2_{y(3.12)}$$

Of course, the last coefficient of semipartial determination on the right of this equation is equal to the coefficient of determination between the dependent variable, y, and the third independent variable, x_3, residualized with respect to the other two independent variables, x_1 and x_2.

This process can be extended to any number of independent variables. One of the advantages of this approach to the decomposition of the coefficient of determination is that it enables us to compare the contributions of sets of variables to explaining the variance in the dependent variable. For example, we might wish to identify the proportion of the variance in the dependent variable explained by three the variables, controlling for the variance in that dependent variable already explained by two other independent variables. We could obtain this result from the following equation:

$$R^2_{y(345.12)} = R^2_{y.12345} - R^2_{y.12}$$

Of course, the incremental contributions of successive variables or sets of variables typically become smaller because these independent variables are usually correlated with the other independent variables.

CHAPTER 22

Testing Simple Hypotheses
Using the F Test

To this point, we have relied solely on the t test to assess the statistical significance of either the simple or partial regression coefficient. However, we can now introduce another statistical test: the F test. As we shall see, the F test is a much more useful statistical test. It can be used to test either simple hypotheses or a variety of compound hypotheses. For example, it can be used to test the significance of either a single regression coefficient or a series of regression coefficients. Consequently, the F test can be substituted for the t test to evaluate the significance of a single regression coefficient. There are many forms of this test; however, for the sake of simplicity, we shall confine ourselves to the F test expressed in terms of the coefficient of determination.

We begin by examining the simplest variant of the F test: the form used to test whether or not a simple regression coefficient is significantly different that zero. In this particular case, the equation for the F ratio is given by:

$$F = \frac{r^2_{yx}}{(1 - r^2_{yx}) \,/\, (N-2)}$$

where r^2_{yx} is the coefficient of determination for the simple regression equation and N refers to the number of observations in the sample. This form of the F test is used to test the following null hypothesis:

$$H_0: \; b_{yx} = 0$$

It is important to note that, although the null hypothesis is stated in terms of the simple regression coefficient, the F test involves only the coefficient of determination associated with that simple regression equation. If the simple regression coefficient between a dependent variable and an independent variable is equal to zero, then the coefficient of determination, which measures the proportion of the variance in the dependent variable accounted for by the independent variable, must also be equal to zero. Of course, due to sampling error, the sample regression coefficient and the sample coefficient of determination may not be equal to zero, even if the population regression coefficient and the population coefficient of determination are equal to zero.

Once the F test value has been computed, it is evaluated with respect to the F distribution. Unfortunately, the F distribution is much more complicated than the t distribution. Like the t distribution, the F distribution is actually a family of distributions. Specifically, the probability density function for the F distribution has two parameters: one for the degrees of freedom in the numerator of the F test and another for the degrees of freedom in the denominator of this test. Therefore, in order to evaluate the statistical significance of any F test, we must compute the appropriate degrees of freedom. In the case of a simple regression equation, the numerator degrees of freedom for the F test is always equal to one because there is only one independent variable in a simple regression equation. Similarly, in the case of a simple regression equation, the denominator degrees of freedom for the F test is equal to the number of observations minus two because two degrees of freedom are expended in computing the parameters of a simple regression equation: one for the regression coefficient and another for the intercept. If the observed F test value is greater than or equal to the critical value of the F distribution with these degrees of freedom, we must reject the null hypothesis that there is no relationship between the variables. It should be noted that the F test value can never be negative because the F test is a ratio of quantities that cannot assume any negative values.

Although it may not be apparent at first, this simple F test is directly related to the t test. Indeed, there is a direct mathematical relationship between the simple regression coefficient and the coefficient of determination for a simple regression equation. Given this fact, we should not be surprised to learn that there is a mathematical relationship between the t test for a simple regression coefficient and the F test for the coefficient of determination of a simple regression equation. Specifically, in this simple case, the F test value is equal to the squared t test value such that:

$$F_{(1, N-2)} = t^2_{(N-2)}$$

Of course, the F test has two subscripts, one for the numerator degrees of freedom and another for the denominator degrees of freedom, whereas the t test has only one.

In order to see the relationship between these two statistical tests, let us consider the regression of public expenditures, y, on economic openness, x_1, in seven major industrial nations. The value of the t test for the significance of this simple regression coefficient can be computed as follows:

$$t = \frac{b_{y1}}{s_b} = \frac{0.731}{0.290} = 2.521$$

Similarly, the value of the F test for the significance of this same regression coefficient can be computed as follows:

$$F = \frac{r^2_{y1}}{(1-r^2_{y1})/(N-2)} = \frac{0.560}{(1-0.560)/(7-2)}$$

$$= \frac{0.560}{0.088} = 6.356$$

It can be seen that the F test value for the simple coefficient of determination is equal to the square of the t test value for the simple regression coefficient. According to the table of critical values for the F distribution with one numerator degree of freedom and 5 denominator degrees of freedom, we require an F test value of 6.61 in order to achieve statistical significance at the conventional 0.05 probability level. Therefore, we cannot reject the null hypothesis of no relationship between the variables. In fact, the exact probability of both the t test value and the F test value is 0.053.

CHAPTER 23

Testing Compound Hypotheses Using the F Test

The real utility of the F test stems from the fact that it can be used to test compound hypotheses. In short, it can be used to test hypotheses in which restrictions are imposed upon several regression coefficients at once. Specifically, the F test can be used to test whether or not all of the partial regression coefficients in a multiple regression equation are equal to zero. For example, we might use the F test to test the following compound hypothesis:

$$H_0: \quad b_{y1.2} = b_{y2.1} = 0$$

In this case, the null hypothesis imposes the restrictions that both of the partial regression coefficients are equal to zero. If both of these partial regression coefficients are equal to zero, it follows that the coefficient of determination for the multiple regression equation containing these two independent is equal to zero. Of course, due to sampling error, the sample coefficient of determination may not be exactly equal to zero, even though the population coefficient of determination is equal to zero. Consequently, the F test is used to determine whether or not we might have obtained a particular nonzero coefficient of determination in the sample by chance, even though the coefficient of determination in the population is zero.

The form of the F test required to test compound hypotheses is slightly more complicated than that used to test a simple hypothesis. Specifically, the form of the F test required to test the hypothesis that all of the partial regression coefficients in a multiple regression equation are equal to zero is given by:

$$F_{(k, N-k-1)} = \frac{R^2_{y.ijk} / k}{(1 - R^2_{y.ijk}) / (N - k - 1)}$$

This form of the F test is similar to the earlier form with only a few differences. First, the coefficient of determination for the simple regression equation is replaced by the coefficient of determination for the multiple regression equation. Second, the coefficient of determination in the numerator is divided by k, the number of independent variables in the regression equation. This quantity did not appear in the F test for the simple regression equation because it was implicitly assumed it was equal to one. Third, the quantity $N - 2$ in the denominator is replaced by the quantity $(N - k - 1)$, the number of observations minus one more than the number of independent variables. In the case of the F test for the simple regression equation, it was implicitly assumed that the number of independent variables was equal to one.

Therefore, the specific F test required to test the compound hypothesis that both partial regression coefficients in a multiple regression equation are equal to zero is given by:

$$F_{(2, N-3)} = \frac{R^2_{y.12} / 2}{(1 - R^2_{y.12}) / (N - 3)}$$

In evaluating the statistical significance of this F test, we employ an F distribution with two numerator degrees of freedom and $N - 3$ denominator degrees of freedom. The numerator has two degrees of freedom because the model being tested has two independent variables. The denominator has $N - 3$ degrees of freedom because three degrees of freedom have been expended in computing the parameters of this multiple regression equation: one for each of the two partial regression coefficients and another for the intercept.

In order to see an application of this form of the F test, let us consider the regression of public expenditures, y, on both economic openness, x_1, and labor organization, x_2. The relevant coefficient of determination is given as follows:

$$R^2_{y.12} = 0.679$$

such that:

$$F_{(2,N-3)} = \frac{0.679 / 2}{(1 - 0.679) / (7 - 3)} = \frac{0.339}{0.080} = 4.237$$

Using the F distribution with two numerator degrees of freedom and four denominator degrees of freedom, we find that we require an F test value of 6.94 in order to achieve statistical significance at the 0.05 probability level. In other words, we cannot reject the null hypothesis that both partial regression coefficients are equal to zero. Indeed, the exact probability of this coefficient of determination is 0.103. Of course, the lack of statistical significance in this particular example is attributable, in large part, to the extremely small sample size.

It can be seen that this equation for the F test is a ratio of some highly interpretable quantities that have been adjusted for their respective degrees of freedom. For example, we can express the F test as follows:

$$F = \frac{\text{Explained Variance / d.f. Expended}}{\text{Unexplained Variance / d.f. Remaining}}$$

First, the coefficient of determination in the numerator of this F test represents the proportion of the variance in the dependent variable explained by the independent variables. This quantity is divided by the number of degrees of freedom expended in estimating the regression coefficients for the independent variables in the multiple regression model. Second, the quantity one minus the coefficient of determination in the denominator of this F test represents the proportion of the variance in the dependent variable that is left unexplained by the independent variables. This quantity is divided by the number of degrees of freedom remaining after estimating the regression coefficients and the intercept of the regression equation.

It must be pointed out there is a fundamental difference between testing a compound hypothesis that two or more partial regression coefficients are equal to zero and testing the separate simple hypotheses that each partial regression coefficient is equal to zero. This fact can be seen from the equation for the relationship between the F test for the compound hypothesis that two partial regression coefficients are equal to zero and the t tests for simple hypotheses that each of these two partial regression coefficients is equal to zero given by:

$$F_{(2,N-3)} = \frac{t_1^2 + t_2^2 + 2t_1 t_2 r_{12}}{2(1-r_{12}^2)}$$

This equation demonstrates that, whenever two independent variables are uncorrelated with one another, the F test is equal to the square of the average of the t tests associated with these two partial regression coefficients. However, whenever the two independent variables are highly correlated, the F test will be much larger than the square of the average of these two t tests.

   This result makes a great deal of intuitive sense when we recall that the standard error of the partial regression coefficient becomes very large whenever an independent variable is highly correlated with the other independent variables in a multiple regression equation. In the case of two highly correlated independent variables, it is possible that neither of them will have a partial regression coefficient that is statistically significant, according to the t test, even though they are both highly related to the dependent variable. In this situation, however, the proportion of variance in the dependent variable explained by both independent variables together may be statistically significant, according to the F test. The relationship between the F test and the t tests in the case of a multiple regression model with two independent variables should alert us to the problems of comparing tests of simple hypotheses involving a single partial regression coefficient and tests of compound hypotheses involving two or more partial regression coefficients.

CHAPTER 24

Testing Hypotheses in
Nested Regression Models

_____

In addition to testing compound hypotheses, the F test can be used to test hypotheses associated with "nested" regression models. Nested hypotheses arise whenever we are interested in comparing two regression equations that are identical except that one contains restrictions that are not imposed on the other. By convention, the regression equation that is free of any restrictions is referred to as the "full" model. Conversely, the regression equation that contains one or more restrictions is referred to as the "restricted" model. Although we can impose different types of restrictions on the restricted model, the most common restriction is simply that one or more partial regression coefficients are equal to zero. In this case, the restricted model becomes a subset of the full model inasmuch as it contains only some of the independent variables contained in the full model. The utility of this application of the F test is that it enables us to evaluate simultaneously the statistical significance of one set of independent variables, controlling for another set independent variables.

It turns out that the forms of the F test that we have used to test simple and compound hypotheses are special cases of a more general form of the F test. Specifically, the general equation for the F test is given by:

$$F = \frac{(R_F^2 - R_R^2) / (k_F - k_R)}{(1 - R_F^2) / (N - k_F - 1)}$$

where R_F^2 is the coefficient of determination for the full model, R_R^2 is the coefficient of determination for the restricted model, k_F is the number of independent variables in the full model, and k_R is the number of independent variables in the restricted model. Of course, N refers to the number of observations in the sample.

The restrictions that we impose on the restricted model are typically that one or more of the partial regression coefficients are equal to zero. Alternatively, we might impose the restrictions that two or more partial regression coefficients are equal to one another. For example, we might wish to test the hypothesis that two independent variables, x_1 and x_2, have no effect on the dependent variable, y, controlling for the effects of a third independent variable, x_3. This hypothesis can be stated in terms of restrictions imposed on the partial regression coefficients of these two variables such that:

$$H_o: \quad b_{y1.23} \quad = \quad b_{y2.13} \quad = \quad 0$$

It is important to note that the subscripts for these partial regression coefficients indicate that the full model contains three independent variables such that:

$$y \quad = \quad ua \quad + \quad x_1 b_{y1.23} \quad + \quad x_2 b_{y2.13} \quad + \quad x_3 b_{y3.12} \quad + \quad e$$

Whenever we impose restrictions on a model that set one or more partial regression coefficients equal to zero, we are effectively deleting these variables from the model. Consequently, the restricted model is simply a subset of the full model inasmuch as it contains only some of the independent variables contained in the full model. For example, in this particular case, the restricted model is given by:

$$y \quad = \quad ua \quad + \quad x_3 b_{y3} \quad + \quad e$$

In short, the *full model* is the regression equation containing *all* of the relevant independent variables. Conversely, the *restricted model* is the regression equation containing all of the relevant independent variables *except* the variable or variables whose statistical significance is being tested. In other words, the restricted model is "restricted" in the sense that it "excludes" one or more variables for the purpose of testing their statistical significance. In effect, we are assessing the statistical significance of one or more independent variables by comparing the variance explained by a full model that includes these variables with the variance explained by a restricted model that excludes them.

The F test required to test the hypothesis that the two partial regression coefficients, $b_{y1.23}$ and $b_{y2.13}$, are equal to zero is given as follows:

$$F = \frac{(R^2_{y.123} - r^2_{y3})/(3-1)}{(1 - R^2_{y.123})/(N-3-1)}$$

Of course, this test is equivalent to testing the null hypothesis that the variance explained in variable y by variables x_1 and x_2, over and above the variance already explained by variable x_3, is equal to zero. In this case, the F test value must be evaluated with two degrees of freedom in the numerator and $N - 4$ degrees of freedom in the denominator in order to determine its probability level. There are two numerator degrees of freedom because the full model requires us to estimate two more partial regression coefficients than the restricted model. Similarly, there are $N - 4$ denominator degrees of freedom because four degrees of freedom are lost in estimating the intercept and the three partial regression coefficients in the full model.

These computations can be demonstrated with a simple example in which we wish to test the hypothesis that economic openness, x_1, and labor organization, x_2, have no effect on public expenditures, y, controlling for the effect of political protest, x_3. The F test for the null hypothesis that these two partial regression coefficients are equal to zero is given by:

$$F = \frac{(R^2_{y.123} - r^2_{y3})/(3-1)}{(1 - R^2_{y.123})/(N-3-1)} = \frac{(0.689 - 0.010)/2}{(1 - 0.689)/3}$$

$$= \frac{0.679/2}{0.311/3} = \frac{0.339}{0.104} = 3.260$$

Given the fact that the F value required for this test to be significant at the 0.05 probability level with two numerator degrees of freedom and three denominator degrees of freedom is 9.55, we cannot reject the null hypothesis that these two partial regression coefficients are equal to zero. Indeed, the exact probability of this F test is 0.18. Once again, the lack of statistical significance is due primarily to the extremely small sample size.

As before, the equation for the F test identifies those factors that will contribute to the significance of any given set of independent variables within a multiple regression equation. For example, we might express the F test as follows:

$$F = \frac{\text{Additional Var. Explained / Additional d.f. Expended}}{\text{Var. Unexplained / d.f. Remaining}}$$

First, the difference between the two coefficients of determination in the numerator of the F test represents the additional variance explained by the full model over and above that already explained by the restricted model. This quantity is equal, of course, to the coefficient of semipartial determination. This coefficient of semipartial determination is divided by the number of additional degrees of freedom expended in the full model over and above the number of degrees of freedom already expended in the restricted model. Second, the quantity one minus the coefficient of determination in the denominator of this F test represents the proportion of the variance in the dependent variable that is not explained by the full model. This quantity is divided by the number of degrees of freedom remaining in the full model after estimating the regression coefficients and the intercept associated with the full model.

It has been noted earlier that a simple variant of the F test can be substituted for the t test to determine the significance of a regression coefficient in a simple regression equation. It should be apparent that this variant of the F test can be substituted for the t test to determine the significance of a single partial regression coefficient in a multiple regression equation. In this case, the restricted model assumes that one of the partial regression coefficients is equal to zero. Specifically, the F test for the significance of a single partial regression coefficient is given by:

$$F = \frac{R_F^2 - R_R^2}{(1 - R_F^2) / (N - k_F - 1)}$$

This simple variant of the F test obtains simply because the numerator degrees of freedom, which is equal to the difference in the number of independent variables in the full and restricted models, is equal to one.

Moreover, there is a mathematical relationship between the F test for the significance of a single partial regression coefficient and the t test for the significance of this partial regression coefficient such that:

$$F_{(1, N-k-1)} = t^2_{(N-k-1)}$$

In short, the value of the F test with one degree of freedom in the numerator and $N - k - 1$ degrees of freedom in the denominator is equal to the squared value of the t test with $N - k - 1$ degrees of freedom, where k is the number of independent variables in the full model and N is the number of observations.

Finally, it must be reiterated that the F test used to evaluate the statistical significance of several partial regression coefficients does not always yield the same results as the t tests for these individual partial regression coefficients. For example, the F test might indicate that three partial regression coefficients are equal to zero, but the t tests for each of these partial regression coefficients might indicate that one of these partial regression coefficients is, in fact, not equal to zero. This might occur whenever one independent variable is marginally significant and the other independent variables being evaluated are not. In these situations, it must be recalled that the F test is being used to evaluate a compound hypothesis that the additional variance explained by adding a series of independent variables to the multiple regression equation simultaneously is not statistically significant. That is not the same as evaluating the simple hypothesis that the additional variable explained by adding one of these independent variables is not statistically significant. There are situations in which we are interested in the aggregate effect of a set of independent variables rather than the separate effects of each of these independent variables.

CHAPTER 25

Testing for Interaction in Multiple Regression

In multiple regression analysis, we make the initial assumption that the effects of the independent variables on the dependent variable are additive. In short, we assume that the dependent variable can be predicted most accurately by a linear function of the independent variables. However, the effects of independent variables on a dependent variable are not always additive. We refer to the presence of nonadditive effects as interaction. *Interaction occurs whenever the effect of an independent variable on a dependent variable is not constant over all of the values of the other independent variables.* Although interaction is a somewhat difficult concept to envision in the abstract, it is not difficult to conceive of situations that would entail interactions between variables. Let us consider, once again, the example of explaining welfare expenditures among seven major industrial nations in terms of economic openness and labor organization. A positive interaction between the independent variables would yield a level of public expenditures among those nations with high levels of both economic openness and labor organization that is higher than we would expect on the basis of the additive effects of these independent variables alone. Conversely, a negative interaction between these independent variables would yield a level of public expenditures among those nations with high levels of both economic openness and labor organization that is lower than we would expect on the basis of the additive effects of these two independent variables.

In order to understand this situation more clearly, we begin with the additive multiple regression model. It will be recalled that the parameters of this particular multiple regression model were given by:

$$\hat{y} = u\,(25.05) + x_1\,(0.452) + x_2\,(0.295)$$

These parameters imply that for every 1 percent increase in economic openness, x_1, holding constant labor organization, x_2, we expect a 0.45 percent increase in public expenditures, y. Similarly, for every 1 percent increase in labor organization, x_2, holding constant economic openness, x_1, we expect a 0.29 percent increase in public expenditures, y. In short, the partial regression coefficients measure the additive effects of each independent variable on the dependent variable.

In order to determine whether or not there is any interaction between economic openness, x_1, and labor organization, x_2, with respect to public expenditures, y, we create an interaction variable. *An interaction variable is any variable that is a product of two or more other variables.* In this particular case, we create an interaction variable, x_3, that is a multiplicative function of the two independent variables, x_1 and x_2, such that:

$$x_{3i} = x_{1i}\,x_{2i}$$

Consequently, the values of this interaction variable are given by the following vector:

$$\mathbf{x}_3 = \begin{bmatrix} x_{31} \\ x_{32} \\ x_{33} \\ x_{34} \\ x_{35} \\ x_{36} \\ x_{37} \end{bmatrix} = \begin{bmatrix} x_{11}\,x_{21} \\ x_{12}\,x_{22} \\ x_{13}\,x_{23} \\ x_{14}\,x_{24} \\ x_{15}\,x_{25} \\ x_{16}\,x_{26} \\ x_{17}\,x_{27} \end{bmatrix} = \begin{bmatrix} (26.8)\,(45.0) \\ (27.4)\,(27.0) \\ (22.6)\,(24.0) \\ (28.9)\,(32.0) \\ (23.0)\,(41.0) \\ (14.8)\,(16.0) \\ (9.7)\,(21.0) \end{bmatrix} = \begin{bmatrix} 1206.0 \\ 739.8 \\ 542.4 \\ 924.8 \\ 943.0 \\ 236.8 \\ 203.7 \end{bmatrix}$$

The values of this interaction variable are not readily interpretable. However, it is evident that the absolute magnitude of the interaction variable depends directly on the absolute magnitude of the two independent variables used to create it. If an observation has large values on both independent variables, it will have a correspondingly large value on the interaction variable. Conversely, if it has small values on both independent variables, it will have a correspondingly small value on the interaction variable. Of course, if an observation has a negative value on one of the two independent variables, it will have a negative value on the interaction variable. However, if it has a negative value on both of the independent variables, it will have a positive value on the interaction variable.

We can test for the presence of interaction between two independent variables with respect to the dependent variable by including the interaction variable in the multiple regression equation with these two independent variables. Specifically, parameters of the multiple regression model with interaction are as follows:

$$\hat{y} = u\,(-12.06) + x_1\,(2.11) + x_2\,(2.01) + x_3\,(-0.07)$$

In order to test for interaction between the two independent variables, x_1 and x_2, with respect to the dependent variable, y, we simply test the statistical significance of the partial regression coefficient of the interaction variable, x_3. Specifically, we test the following null hypothesis:

$$H_0: b_{y3.12} = 0$$

In this particular case, we can test the significance of the partial regression coefficient for this single interaction variable using either the t test or the F test. The results of the F test for the significance of this partial regression coefficient for the interaction variable are presented as follows:

$$F = \frac{(R^2_{y.123} - R^2_{y.12})}{(1 - R^2_{y.123})\,/\,(N-4)} = \frac{(0.784 - 0.679)}{(1 - 0.784)\,/\,3}$$

$$= \frac{0.105\,/\,1}{0.216\,/\,3} = \frac{0.105}{0.072} = 1.46$$

As the coefficients of determination for these two multiple regression models indicate, the full model that includes the interaction variable explains more of the variance in the dependent variable than the restricted model that excludes this variable. Specifically, the coefficient of determination for the model with interaction explains 78 percent of the variance in public expenditures, whereas the model without interaction explains only 68 percent of the variance in this variable. However, this increment in explained variance is not statistically significant at the conventional 0.05 probability level, due primarily to the extremely small sample size.

Of course, it must be noted that the possibilities for interaction among the independent variables in a regression model increase geometrically with increases in the number of independent variables. In a regression model with only two independent variables, there is only one possible interaction variable. However, in regression models with three independent variables, there are four possible interaction variables. Specifically, it is possible to construct three first-order interaction variables that are products of each pair of independent variables as well as one second-order interaction variable that is the product of all three independent variables. Moreover, in a regression model with four independent variables, there are 11 possible interaction variables: six first-order interaction variables, four second-order interaction variables, and one third-order interaction variable. Whenever we have a large number of interaction variables, we can test for the statistical significance of all of them simultaneously using the F test. In other words, we can compare a full model that includes all of the interaction variables with a restricted model that excludes all of them. Alternatively, we can seek to identify statistically significant interactions among sets of independent variables by examining the t tests for the partial regression coefficients of these interaction variables. As a practical matter, we do not usually test for interactions among independent variables unless we have some theoretical basis for suspecting the presence of interaction between particular sets of variables.

Finally, we must understand that the presence of interaction in a multiple regression model greatly complicates the interpretation of the partial regression coefficients. Indeed, whenever there is a statistically significant interaction in a multiple regression model, the net effect of any independent variable on the dependent variable consists of the sum of its main effect and its interaction effect. This interaction effect is, in turn, determined by the level of the other independent variable or variables used to create the relevant interaction variables. For example, the net effect of economic openness on public expenditures is equal to the sum of its main effect, $b_{y1.23}$, and its interaction effect, given by the product of the partial regression coefficient for the interaction between economic openness and labor organization and the level of labor organization, $b_{y3.12}\, x_1$. In short, the expected change in the dependent variable produced by a one unit change in this independent variable is contingent upon the level of the other independent variable. For example, the negative partial regression coefficient for the interaction between economic openness and labor organization means indicates that a one unit increase in economic openness will produce a smaller increase in public expenditures whenever the level of labor organization is high than it will whenever the level of labor organization is low. The difficulties entailed in interpreting the partial regression coefficients in multiple regression models with interaction provide us with ample motivation for conducting the statistical tests required to discount this possibility. Fortunately, statistically significant interactions among continuous independent variables are not all that commonplace in empirical research.

CHAPTER 26

Nonlinear Relationships and Variable Transformations

It will be recalled that simple regression analysis assumes, from the very outset, that the relationship between two variables is at least approximately linear. More precisely, regression analysis estimates the parameters of the linear regression equation that best describes the relationship between two variables. In this case, "best" is defined in terms of the linear regression equation that minimizes the sum of squared errors of prediction and, therefore, maximizes the coefficient of determination. Regression analysis employs a linear function to describe the relationship between two variables because linear functions are simpler than most other mathematical equations. The principle of parsimony in science dictates that, other things being equal, simple explanations are preferable to complex ones. Therefore, whenever two regression equations, one linear and the other nonlinear, explain the same amount of variance in a dependent variable, we should choose the linear regression equation because it is simpler than the nonlinear regression equation. Of course, some empirical relationships are inherently nonlinear and can be described only very imprecisely by a linear regression equation.

Before examining various types of nonlinear relationships and how they might be examined using regression analysis, it is important to understand the fundamental difference between linear and nonlinear relationships. Simply stated, a linear relationship is one in which the expected change in the dependent variable associated with a given change in the independent variable is constant for all values of the

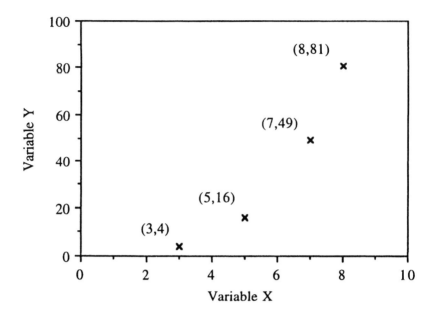

Figure 26.1. Relationship between Variable X and and Variable Y

independent variable. *Conversely, a nonlinear relationship is one in which the expected change in the dependent variable associated with a given change in the independent variable is not constant for all values of the independent variable.* For example, when the value of the independent variable is relatively small, a small change in that variable might yield only a small change in the dependent variable. However, when the value of the independent variable is relatively large, a small change in that variable might yield a large change in the dependent variable. Since the expected change in the dependent variable associated with a given change in the independent variable is not constant over all of the values of the independent variable, we must conclude that the relationship between them is nonlinear.

The linear regression model can readily be adapted to accommodate a variety of different nonlinear relationships. Specifically, nonlinear relationships can be incorporated into the linear regression model simply by performing nonlinear transformations on the variables in order to render the relationship between them more linear.

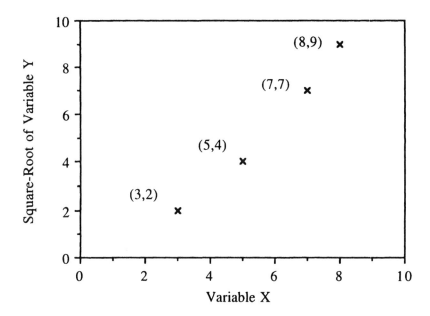

Figure 26.2.   Relationship between Variable X and the
Square Root of Variable Y

We can demonstrate the utility of such a variable transformation using a simple and somewhat artificial example. Consider the relationship between the two variables presented in Figure 26.1. Obviously, the relationship between variable x and variable y is nonlinear. We might use a linear regression equation to describe the relationship between these two variables, but such a regression equation would not explain the variance in the dependent variable as well as a regression equation that models the form of the nonlinearity between these two variables. In this somewhat contrived example, we can transform the nonlinear relationship into a much more linear relationship by imposing a nonlinear transformation on the dependent variable. In this particular case, we can obtain a more linear relationship between these two variables by simply taking the square roots of the values of variable y. The relationship between variable x and the square root of variable y is presented in Figure 26.2.

Although the square root transformation is based on a familiar mathematical function and is convenient in many applications, it is not the most common nonlinear transformation employed in regression analysis.   Instead, the most common nonlinear transformation employed in regression analysis involves the natural logarithmic function.   For example, we might reduce the degree of nonlinearity between two variables by transforming the independent variable using the natural logarithm, such that:

$$y_i = a + b\tilde{x}_i + e_i$$

where

$$\tilde{x}_i = \log(x_i)$$

Alternatively, we might subject the dependent variable to a logarithmic transformation.   Moreover, it is possible to subject both the dependent and independent variables to the same nonlinear transformation.

Indeed, a linear regression equation in which all of the variables have been subjected to logarithmic transformations can be used to estimate the parameters of multiplicative regression model.   For example, it is possible to estimate the parameters of a multiplicative regression model using the linear regression model simply by taking the logarithms of each variable as follows:

$$y_i = a x_i^b e_i$$

such that:

$$\log(y_i) = \log(a) + b\log(x_i) + \log(e_i)$$

In other words, we can regress the logarithm of variable y on the logarithm of variable x.   The value of b in the multiplicative regression model can be obtained directly from the regression coefficient in the linear regression model.   The value of a in the multiplicative regression model is obtained by taking the antilogarithm of the intercept in the linear regression model.

Finally, it must be noted that both the square root transformation and the logarithmic transformation are what are known as monotonic transformations.   In a monotonic transformation, there is an ordinal relationship between the values of the original variable and the values of the transformed variable.   It is possible, of course, to employ nonmonotonic transformations in order to render the relationship between two variables more linear. These transformations are especially appropriate whenever there is a curvilinear relationship between two variables such that the direction of the relationship between them changes at some point. The most common nonmonotonic transformation involves the quadratic function. For example, we can regress a dependent variable on two variables that represent a quadratic function as follows:

$$y_i = a + b_{yx} x_i + b_{yv} v_i + e_i$$

where

$$v_i = x_i^2$$

Although there are ostensibly two independent variables in this regression equation, the second independent variable is a strict mathematical function of the first independent variable. Depending on the signs of the regression coefficients, a quadratic equation can be used to model either a ∪-shaped or a ∩-shaped relationship between a dependent variable and an independent variable.

CHAPTER 27

Regression Analysis with Dummy Variables

Up to this point, we have implicitly assumed that all of the variables in our regression models are continuous. However, sometimes we are interested in using independent variables that are categorical rather than continuous. A categorical variable is one that consists of a series of categories that are both exhaustive and mutually exclusive such that each observation is assigned to one and no more than one category. There are many variables in social science research, such as gender, ethnicity, and marital status, that are inherently categorical. It turns out that categorical variables can be used as independent variables in regression analysis without much difficulty. Indeed, regression analysis with categorical independent variables provides results that are identical with those obtained from a statistical technique known as *analysis of variance*.

Specifically, it is possible to conduct an analysis of variance using the regression model by creating special variables to represent the categories of our categorical variables. The simplest and most common method of creating variables to represent categories is known as *dummy variable analysis*. In order to employ this technique, it is necessary to create a series of binary variables that identify whether or not each observation is a member of a specific category or group. *A binary variable is a variable that is coded either as a one or as a zero.* If an observation is classified as a member of a particular category, then it is coded as a one on the binary variable representing that category. Otherwise, this observation is coded as a zero on this binary variable.

In order to see how dummy variables are created, let us consider the example of gender. We shall assume that everyone in our sample can be classified as either a man or a woman. In short, we will assume that this categorical variable, composed of only two categories, is both exhaustive and mutually exclusive. In this case, we might construct a binary variable for men in which every man is assigned a one and every woman is assigned a zero. Alternatively, we might construct a binary variable for women in which every woman is assigned a one and every man is assigned a zero. It is important to note that, given the information contained in one of these binary variables, the information contained in the other binary variable is redundant. This situation arises because the binary variables representing each of these two categories are mathematical functions of one another. Any observation coded with a zero on one binary variable must be coded with a one on the other binary variable and vice versa.

This simple fact creates a computational problem with respect to using two or more binary variables that are mathematical functions of one another in the same regression model. It will be recalled that the regression equation almost invariably includes an intercept. Indeed, almost all computer programs that perform regression analysis automatically construct a binary variable consisting entirely of ones to represent the intercept. The binary variable representing the intercept is then treated as an independent variable in the model. This convention creates a computational problem if we attempt to include two or more binary variables that are mathematical functions of one another in a regression model that includes an intercept. The problem arises because the intercept will be an exact linear function of the binary variables representing the categories of this categorical variable. In this situation, there will be exact multicollinearity between the intercept and these binary variables. As a result, the computer program will not be able to obtain least-squares estimates of the parameters of the multiple regression equation. More specifically, the matrix of correlations among the independent binary variables, including the binary variable representing the intercept, will be singular and it will not be possible to compute its inverse.

This problem can be readily circumvented but only at the cost of complicating the analysis. The solution involves the use of dummy variables in the regression model. *Dummy variable analysis involves a regression model with binary variables representing all but one of the categories of each categorical variable.* In other words, one of the categories of the categorical variable must be excluded from the analysis. For example, we can use either the binary variable for men or the binary variable for women in a regression model, but we cannot use them both at the same time whenever there is an intercept in the model. In short, dummy variables analysis allows us to use binary variables, representing the categories of a categorical variable, in a regression model as long as we exclude one of the categories from the analysis. Once a category has been excluded from the analysis and binary variables have been constructed for each of the remaining categories, it is a simple matter to use these binary variables in a regression model in order to conduct an analysis of variance.

Let us consider a simple empirical example in which we wish to examine the effects of gender on the incomes of six individuals: three men and three women. If men are defined as the excluded category, then a regression model can be constructed using a single dummy variable, which represents women, as follows:

$$\mathbf{y} = \mathbf{u}a + \mathbf{x}b + \mathbf{e}$$

where the vectors are given as follows:

$$
\begin{bmatrix} 27 \\ 24 \\ 21 \\ 21 \\ 18 \\ 15 \end{bmatrix}
=
\begin{bmatrix} 1 \\ 1 \\ 1 \\ 1 \\ 1 \\ 1 \end{bmatrix} a
+
\begin{bmatrix} 0 \\ 0 \\ 0 \\ 1 \\ 1 \\ 1 \end{bmatrix} b
+
\begin{bmatrix} e_1 \\ e_2 \\ e_3 \\ e_4 \\ e_5 \\ e_6 \end{bmatrix}
$$

The values of the intercept and the regression coefficient for this equation can be obtained using ordinary least-squares estimation procedures. In this simple example, these results are obtained from the familiar equations for the simple regression coefficient and the intercept as follows:

$$\text{Cov}(x,y) = \frac{1}{N}(\mathbf{x}'\mathbf{y} - \bar{\mathbf{x}}'\bar{\mathbf{y}}) = \frac{1}{N}\sum x_i y_i - \bar{x}\,\bar{y}$$

$$= \frac{1}{6}(54) = 10.5 = 9 - 10.5 = -1.50$$

$$Var(x) \; = \; \frac{1}{N} \, (x'x - \bar{x}'\bar{x}) \; = \; \frac{1}{N} \Sigma x_i^2 - \bar{x}^2$$

$$= \; \frac{1}{6} \, (3) - 0.25 \; = \; 0.50 - 0.25 \; = \; 0.25$$

such that:

$$b \; = \; \frac{Cov(x,y)}{Var(x)} \; = \; \frac{-1.50}{0.25} \; = \; -6.00$$

$$a \; = \; \bar{y} - b\bar{x} \; = \; 21 - (-6.00)(0.50) \; = \; 21 + 3 \; = \; 24$$

Using these least-squares estimates of the simple regression coefficient and the intercept, the vector of predicted scores from this regression equation is given as follows:

$$\hat{y} \; = \; u \, (24) + x \, (-6) \; = \; \begin{bmatrix} 24 \\ 24 \\ 24 \\ 24 \\ 24 \\ 24 \end{bmatrix} + \begin{bmatrix} 0 \\ 0 \\ 0 \\ -6 \\ -6 \\ -6 \end{bmatrix} \; = \; \begin{bmatrix} 24 \\ 24 \\ 24 \\ 18 \\ 18 \\ 18 \end{bmatrix}$$

It is possible to interpret both the intercept and the regression coefficient of a regression model with dummy variables. It will be recalled that the intercept of a simple regression equation is equal to the expected value of the dependent variable whenever the value of the independent variable is equal to zero. Therefore, the intercept corresponds to the mean on the dependent variable for the observations in the excluded category. In this case, the intercept indicates that the three men in this analysis have average incomes of $24,000. Similarly, the regression coefficient in a simple regression equation represents the expected change in the dependent variable associated with a one unit change in the independent variable. In dummy variable analysis, the regression coefficient represents the effect on the dependent variable of being in the category represented by the dummy variable instead of being in the excluded category represented by the intercept. In this case, the regression coefficient indicates that the women in the analysis have average incomes that are $6,000 less than those of the men.

Of course, it is possible to compute the errors of prediction in the usual manner such that:

$$
\mathbf{e} = \mathbf{y} - \hat{\mathbf{y}} =
\begin{bmatrix} 27 \\ 24 \\ 21 \\ 21 \\ 18 \\ 15 \end{bmatrix}
-
\begin{bmatrix} 24 \\ 24 \\ 24 \\ 18 \\ 18 \\ 18 \end{bmatrix}
=
\begin{bmatrix} 3 \\ 0 \\ -3 \\ 3 \\ 0 \\ -3 \end{bmatrix}
$$

Finally, it is possible to assess the adequacy of this model by computing the coefficient of determination in the usual manner as follows:

$$
\text{Var}(e) = \frac{1}{N}(\mathbf{e}'\mathbf{e}) = \frac{1}{N}\sum e_i^2 = \frac{1}{6}(36) = 6.00
$$

$$
\text{Var}(y) = \frac{1}{N}(\mathbf{y}'\mathbf{y} - \bar{\mathbf{y}}'\bar{\mathbf{y}}) = \frac{1}{N}\sum y_i^2 - \bar{y}^2
$$

$$
= \frac{1}{6}(2{,}736) - 441 = 456 - 441 = 15
$$

such that:

$$
r_{yx}^2 = 1 - \left(\frac{\text{Var}(e)}{\text{Var}(y)} \right) = 1 - \left(\frac{6.00}{15.00} \right)
$$

$$
= 1 - 0.400 = 0.600
$$

The coefficient of determination for a regression model with dummy variables can be interpreted in terms of the proportion of the variance in the dependent variable that is explained by the categorical variable. In this case, the dummy variable for gender explains 60.0 percent of the variance in income.

CHAPTER 28

One-Way Analysis of Variance Using the Regression Model

An analysis of variance model with just one categorical variable is referred to as a one-way analysis of variance model. Although one-way analysis of variance models are limited to only one categorical variable, this variable can comprise any number of categories. In other words, the categorical variable does not have to be a simple dichotomy. In fact, many categorical variables are not dichotomies. For example, marital status is often treated as a dichotomous variable: one is either married or single. However, the category of single includes individuals who are widowed and divorced as well as those who have never been married. Similarly, minority group status is sometimes treated as a dichotomous variable: one is either a minority or not. However, the category of minority group member includes individuals from two large but very different minority groups: African-Americans and Hispanic-Americans. If we are interested in comparing the effects of different types of minority group status on income, we should probably differentiate between African-Americans and Hispanic-Americans.

It is a simple matter to conduct a one-way analysis of variance in which the categorical variable has more than two categories using a regression model with dummy variables. In order to conduct such an analysis, we simply create binary variables to represent all but one of the categories of the categorical variable. In short, we must always exclude one of the categories of categorical variable from the analysis. From a purely statistical point of view, it does not matter which category we exclude. However, the results of our analysis will be

somewhat easier to interpret if we choose to exclude the category that
serves, in some sense, as the comparison group for the other categories. For example, in a dummy variable regression analysis of the
effects of minority group status on income, we might choose to
exclude the category representing the dominant group so that the
partial regression coefficients measure the effects of being a member
of a minority group instead of the dominant group.

We can illustrate the utility of using a regression model with
dummy variables to perform a one-way analysis of variance, in the
case of a categorical variable with more than two categories, with a
simple example. Let us consider a simple hypothetical example in
which we wish to examine the effects of minority group status on
income within a sample of eight individuals. In this example, the first
four individuals are white-Anglos, the next two individuals are
African-Americans, and the last two individuals are Hispanic-
Americans. If white-Anglos are chosen as the excluded category, then
a regression model can be constructed using two dummy variables:
x_1, representing those individuals who are African-Americans, and x_2,
representing those individuals who are Hispanic-Americans. This
multiple regression model with two dummy variables can be expressed
as follows:

$$y = ua + x_1 b_{y1.2} + x_2 b_{y2.1} + e$$

where the vectors are given as follows:

$$\begin{bmatrix} 22 \\ 24 \\ 26 \\ 28 \\ 20 \\ 18 \\ 22 \\ 30 \end{bmatrix} = \begin{bmatrix} 1 \\ 1 \\ 1 \\ 1 \\ 1 \\ 1 \\ 1 \\ 1 \end{bmatrix} a + \begin{bmatrix} 0 \\ 0 \\ 0 \\ 0 \\ 1 \\ 1 \\ 0 \\ 0 \end{bmatrix} b_{y1.2} + \begin{bmatrix} 0 \\ 0 \\ 0 \\ 0 \\ 0 \\ 0 \\ 1 \\ 1 \end{bmatrix} b_{y2.1} + \begin{bmatrix} e_1 \\ e_2 \\ e_3 \\ e_4 \\ e_5 \\ e_6 \\ e_7 \\ e_8 \end{bmatrix}$$

As before, the values of the intercept and the two partial regression
coefficients for this equation can be obtained using ordinary least-
squares estimation procedures such that:

$$y = u (25.00) + x_1 (-6.00) + x_2 (-4.00) + e$$

These coefficients can be interpreted in a relatively straightforward manner. The intercept, a, represents the mean income for individuals in the excluded category: white-Anglos. Similarly, the partial regression coefficient, $b_{y1.2}$, represents the effect on income of being an African-American instead of being a white-Anglo. Similarly, the partial regression coefficient, $b_{y2.1}$, represents the effect on income of being a Hispanic-American instead of being a white-Anglo. In this case, the expected or mean income for each minority group can be computed easily by adding the partial regression coefficient for the dummy variable representing that group to the intercept representing the dominant group.

Once we have obtained the coefficient of determination for this regression equation, we can test the hypothesis that the mean incomes of the two minority groups are equal to the mean income of the dominant group. This hypothesis is equivalent to the null hypothesis that both of the regression coefficients are equal to zero in the population:

$$H_0 : b_{y1.2} = b_{y2.1} = 0$$

This null hypothesis can be tested using the appropriate form of the F test as follows:

$$F = \frac{R_{y.12}^2 / k_f}{(1 - R_{y.12}^2) / (N - k_f - 1)}$$

$$= \frac{0.692 / 2}{(1 - 0.692) / (8 - 2 - 1)} = \frac{0.346}{0.062} = 5.58$$

Based on this result, with two numerator and five denominator degrees of freedom, we must reject the null hypothesis at the conventional 0.05 probability level. In other words, the dummy variables representing membership in these two minority groups have a statistically significant effect on income.

Another important use of the analysis of variance model is that it allows us to determine whether or not there are significant differences between two or more groups with respect to a dependent variable. For example, we might wish to determine whether or not there are significant differences between African-Americans and Hispanic-Americans in terms of their incomes. We know that the partial regression coefficients for the dummy variables representing these two categories are different, but we do not know whether or not this difference is statistically significant. Specifically, we might wish to test the null hypothesis that the partial regression coefficients for these two categories are equal such that:

$$H_0 : b_{y1.2} = b_{y2.1}$$

It must be noted that the statistical test required to test whether or not two or more partial regression coefficients are equal to one another is not the same as the test required to test whether or not two or more partial regression coefficients are equal to zero.

If the partial regression coefficients for the dummy variables representing two categories of a single categorical variable are equal to one another, then these dummy variables can be combined into a single dummy variable with a single regression coefficient as follows:

$$\mathbf{y} = \mathbf{u}a + \mathbf{x_1}b_{y1.2} + \mathbf{x_2}b_{y2.1} + \mathbf{e}$$

$$= \mathbf{u}a + (\mathbf{x_1} + \mathbf{x_2})b_{y(1+2)} + \mathbf{e}$$

$$= \mathbf{u}a + \mathbf{x_3}b_{y3} + \mathbf{e}$$

If the null hypothesis is correct, a simple regression model with one dummy variable, x_3, representing the sum of the two dummy variables, x_1 and x_2, should explain as much variance in the dependent variable, y, as a multiple regression model with two dummy variables, x_1 and x_2.

In order to test the null hypothesis that the partial regression coefficients for these two dummy variables are equal to one another, we must compare the full model, which includes these two dummy variables, with a restricted model, which includes a single dummy variable that represents the sum of these two dummy variables. In this case, the single dummy variable represents minority group status in general. This regression model with a single dummy variable can be expressed as follows:

$$y = ua + x_3 b_{y3} + e$$

where the vectors are given as follows:

$$\begin{bmatrix} 22 \\ 24 \\ 26 \\ 28 \\ 20 \\ 18 \\ 22 \\ 30 \end{bmatrix} = \begin{bmatrix} 1 \\ 1 \\ 1 \\ 1 \\ 1 \\ 1 \\ 1 \\ 1 \end{bmatrix} a + \begin{bmatrix} 0 \\ 0 \\ 0 \\ 0 \\ 1 \\ 1 \\ 1 \\ 1 \end{bmatrix} b_{y3} + \begin{bmatrix} e_1 \\ e_2 \\ e_3 \\ e_4 \\ e_5 \\ e_6 \\ e_7 \\ e_8 \end{bmatrix}$$

The values of both the intercept and the simple regression coefficient for this equation can be obtained using standard least-squares estimation procedures such that:

$$y = u(25.00) + x_3(-5.00) + e$$

Given the coefficients of determination for both the full and restricted models, we can test the null hypothesis that the mean incomes of the two minority groups are equal using the appropriate form of the F test as follows:

$$F = \frac{(R^2_{y.12} - r^2_{y3})/(k_f - k_r)}{(1 - R^2_{y.12})/(N - k_f - 1)}$$

$$= \frac{(0.692 - 0.641)/(2 - 1)}{(1 - 0.692)/(8 - 2 - 1)} = \frac{0.051}{0.062} = 0.82$$

Based on this result, with one and five degrees of freedom, we fail to reject the null hypothesis at the conventional 0.05 probability level. In other words, the difference in the effects of the dummy variables representing membership in these two minority groups on income is not statistically significant.

CHAPTER 29

Two-Way Analysis of Variance Using the Regression Model

The analysis of variance model can be extended to situations involving two or more categorical independent variables. These more complex analyses of variance can be performed using regression models with dummy variables. In order to understand the logic of these models, we can examine the case of two categorical independent variables. An analysis of variance with two independent variables is referred to as a two-way analysis of variance. Of course, this model can easily be extended to handle additional categorical independent variables. In any event, the approach is similar to that employed in the simple one-way analysis of variance. *In a two-way analysis of variance using regression analysis with dummy variables, binary variables are created to represent all but one of the categories of each categorical independent variable.*

Let us consider a simple example similar to the one that we examined in the case of a one-way analysis of variance. Specifically, we can examine the effects of two categorical independent variables, gender and minority group status, on income. For the sake of simplicity, let us assume that we have four men and four women and that two of the men and two of the women are minorities. According to the conventions of dummy variable regression analysis, we must create a dummy variable for one category of each categorical variable and exclude the other category. For example, we can create a dummy variable, x_1, for those four individuals who are women so that the four men are the excluded category on this categorical variable representing gender. Similarly, we can create another dummy variable, x_2, for those four individuals who are minorities so that the four individuals who are not minorities are the excluded category on this categorical variable representing minority group status.

In order to perform a two-way analysis of variance using regression analysis with dummy variables, we simply estimate the parameters of a regression model that contains two dummy variables as independent variables such that:

$$y = ua + x_1 b_{y1.2} + x_2 b_{y2.1} + e$$

where the vectors contain the following values:

$$
\begin{bmatrix} 21 \\ 27 \\ 23 \\ 25 \\ 19 \\ 21 \\ 15 \\ 17 \end{bmatrix}
=
\begin{bmatrix} 1 \\ 1 \\ 1 \\ 1 \\ 1 \\ 1 \\ 1 \\ 1 \end{bmatrix} a
+
\begin{bmatrix} 0 \\ 0 \\ 0 \\ 0 \\ 1 \\ 1 \\ 1 \\ 1 \end{bmatrix} b_{y1.2}
+
\begin{bmatrix} 1 \\ 0 \\ 1 \\ 0 \\ 1 \\ 0 \\ 1 \\ 0 \end{bmatrix} b_{y2.1}
+
\begin{bmatrix} e_1 \\ e_2 \\ e_3 \\ e_4 \\ e_5 \\ e_6 \\ e_7 \\ e_8 \end{bmatrix}
$$

It is important to remember that there are two excluded categories in a two-way analysis of variance using a regression model with dummy variables. In this particular case, the excluded categories are men and nonminorities. *Therefore, the intercept in a two-way analysis of variance is interpreted as the expected value of those cases in both excluded groups.* In this case, for example, the intercept is the expected value of those individuals who were nonminority men. *Similarly, each partial regression coefficient in a two-way analysis of variance represents the effect of each categorical independent variable on the dependent variable, controlling for the effect of the other categorical independent variables, expressed as a deviation from the expected value for the excluded category.*

The application of ordinary least-squares estimation procedures to the dummy variable regression model for these data yields the following intercept and partial regression coefficients:

$$\hat{y} = u (25.5) + x_1 (-6) + x_2 (-3)$$

The intercept for this model indicates that the expected or mean income for nonminority men, the excluded category, is $25,500. The partial regression coefficient for the binary variable representing women, $b_{y1.2}$, indicates that the effect of being a woman instead of a man, controlling for the effects of minority group status, is to reduce income by $6,000. Similarly, the partial regression coefficient for the binary minority group variable, $b_{y2.1}$, indicates that the effect of being a minority group member instead of a member of the nonminority group, controlling for the effects of gender, is to reduce income by $3,000.

The results of this two-way analysis of variance using a regression model with dummy variables enable us to predict the incomes of the four different "groups" of individuals defined by the gender and minority group status variables. Specifically, predicted incomes for each group are obtained directly from the parameters of the regression model as follows:

$$\hat{y} = \begin{bmatrix} 25.5 \\ 25.5 \\ 25.5 \\ 25.5 \\ 25.5 \\ 25.5 \\ 25.5 \\ 25.5 \end{bmatrix} + \begin{bmatrix} 0 \\ 0 \\ 0 \\ 0 \\ -6 \\ -6 \\ -6 \\ -6 \end{bmatrix} + \begin{bmatrix} -3 \\ 0 \\ -3 \\ 0 \\ -3 \\ 0 \\ -3 \\ 0 \end{bmatrix} = \begin{bmatrix} 22.5 \\ 25.5 \\ 22.5 \\ 25.5 \\ 16.5 \\ 19.5 \\ 16.5 \\ 19.5 \end{bmatrix}$$

In other words, we begin with the predicted value of being a nonminority male and subtract the effects of being a woman or a minority or both. For example, the expected income of a minority women is $16,500. This represents the expected income of nonminority men minus the effect of being a woman and the effect of being a minority.

The coefficient of determination for this model, which is obtained in the usual manner, is 0.804. In other words, 80.4 percent of the variance in the income of these eight individuals can be explained by gender and race. It is important to note that, in this particular case, the two categorical variables, gender and minority group status, are orthogonal, such that:

$$r_{12} = 0$$

These two categorical independent variables are uncorrelated in this particular example because there are an equal number of individuals in each of the four groups: two nonminority men, two minority men, two nonminority women, and two minority women. Categorical independent variables will be orthogonal whenever there are an equal number of observations in each category.

It can be shown that, whenever two or more categorical independent variables are uncorrelated with one another, the coefficient of determination for all of the independent variables together is equal to the sum of the coefficients of determination for each of the variables separately. For example, using regression models with dummy variables to perform separate one-way analyses of variance of these data, it turns out that minority group status alone explains 16.1 percent of the variance in income, whereas gender alone explains another 64.3 percent. Consequently, this coefficient of determination for the regression model with two dummy variables can be partitioned into two orthogonal components such that:

$$R^2_{y.12} = r^2_{y1} + r^2_{y2}$$

$$0.804 = 0.161 + 0.643$$

In other words, a two-way analysis of variance model with orthogonal independent variables permits a decomposition of the total explained variance in a dependent variable into the variance explained by each independent categorical variable separately. This property of analysis of variance with orthogonal variables is so useful that experimental researchers often assign the same number of cases to each experimental condition so they can partition the explained variance in this manner. This approach is known in experimental research as a *balanced design*. Moreover, if two categorical variables are uncorrelated with one another, the partial regression coefficients obtained from the two-way analysis of variance will be equal to the simple regression coefficients obtained from the separate one-way analyses of variance.

It is important to realize that most analyses of nonexperimental data will involve independent variables that are nonorthogonal or correlated. In most case, there will be different numbers of observations in the categories of each categorical variable. For example, in a random sample of the population, we would not expect to find an equal number of minorities and nonminorities. Indeed, we would not even expect to find exactly the same number of men as women in such a sample. Whenever two or more categorical independent variables are correlated with one another, it is not possible to partition the variance explained by each of these variables into orthogonal components. In these cases, we can only partition the variance in a dependent variable in terms of the incremental contributions of variables controlling for the contributions of prior variables. For example, we can determine the proportion of the variance in the dependent variable explained by a given independent variable that is not already explained by other independent variable or variables. This can be achieved by using the coefficient of semipartial determination.

CHAPTER 30

Testing for Interaction
in Analysis of Variance

The regression model, even one employing dummy variables, assumes that the effects of the independent variables on the dependent variable are additive. However, in the presence of interaction, these effects will not be strictly additive. For example, in the dummy variable regression of income on gender and minority group status, interaction would be present if the effect of gender on income was not the same for both minorities and nonminorities. As in the case of multiple regression with continuous variables, we can test for the presence of interaction using interaction variables that are multiplicative functions of the independent variables. These interaction variables also enable us to estimate the effects on the dependent variable of any interaction between the independent variables. In analysis of variance models, of course, both the independent variables and the interaction variables are dummy variables.

In order to understand this problem more clearly, let us consider, once again, the dummy variable regression model required to perform a two-way analysis of variance of income in terms of gender and minority group status. It will be recalled that the parameters of this additive model were given by:

$$\hat{y} \;=\; \mathbf{u}\,(25.5) \;+\; \mathbf{x_1}\,(-6) \;+\; \mathbf{x_2}\,(-3)$$

The intercept indicates that the average income of nonminority men, the compound excluded category in this analysis, is \$25,500. The partial regression coefficient for the dummy variable representing women, x_1, indicates that women can be expected to earn \$6,000 less than men, controlling for the effects of minority group status. Similarly, the partial regression coefficient for the dummy variable representing minorities, x_2, indicates that minorities can be expected to earn \$3,000 less than nonminorities, controlling for the effects of gender. It is important to note that, if there is no interaction between gender and minority group status with respect to income, the effects on income of being both a woman and a minority are strictly additive. Consequently, minority women can be expected to earn \$9,000 less than nonminority men.

Although this additive model provides fairly accurate predictions of the incomes of these eight individuals, it is possible that the effects of gender and minority group status on income are not strictly additive. In short, we might be able to explain more of the variance in income among these eight individuals with the inclusion of an interaction variable that is a multiplicative function of the gender variable and the minority group status variable. This interaction variable would consist of a binary vector that contains a one only for those individuals who are both women and minorities. Consequently, we must estimate the parameters of a multiple regression model that includes the dummy variable representing women, x_1, the dummy variable representing minorities, x_2, and the dummy interaction variable, x_3, as follows:

$$\mathbf{y} = \mathbf{u}a + \mathbf{x_1}b_{y1.23} + \mathbf{x_2}b_{y2.13} + \mathbf{x_3}b_{y3.12} + \mathbf{e}$$

where the vectors contains the following values:

$$
\begin{bmatrix} 21 \\ 27 \\ 23 \\ 25 \\ 19 \\ 21 \\ 17 \\ 15 \end{bmatrix}
=
\begin{bmatrix} 1 \\ 1 \\ 1 \\ 1 \\ 1 \\ 1 \\ 1 \\ 1 \end{bmatrix} a
+
\begin{bmatrix} 0 \\ 0 \\ 0 \\ 0 \\ 1 \\ 1 \\ 1 \\ 1 \end{bmatrix} b_{y1.23}
+
\begin{bmatrix} 1 \\ 0 \\ 1 \\ 0 \\ 1 \\ 0 \\ 1 \\ 0 \end{bmatrix} b_{y2.13}
+
\begin{bmatrix} 0 \\ 0 \\ 0 \\ 0 \\ 1 \\ 0 \\ 1 \\ 0 \end{bmatrix} b_{y3.12}
+
\begin{bmatrix} e_1 \\ e_2 \\ e_3 \\ e_4 \\ e_5 \\ e_6 \\ e_7 \\ e_8 \end{bmatrix}
$$

In other words, this model asserts that the income of each individual is the result of the effect of being a woman, the effect of being a minority, and the effect of being both a woman and a minority.

The application of ordinary least-squares estimation procedures to the multiple regression model for these data yields the following intercept and partial regression coefficients:

$$\hat{y} = (26) + X_1(-7) + X_2(-4) + X_3(2)$$

Of course, whenever there is significant interaction among the independent variables, a regression model that includes these interaction variables will yield different partial regression coefficients for the independent variables than a strictly additive regression model that does not include these interaction variables.

Given these results, we can test whether or not the interaction variable in this model is statistically significant. In this simple case, the statistical significance of the single interaction variable can be tested using either the t test or the F test. In order to test for interaction in this empirical example using the F test, we compare a full model that includes the interaction variable, as well as the two independent variables, with a restricted model that excludes this interaction variable. The coefficient of determination for the full model with the interaction variable is 0.906, whereas the coefficient of determination for the restricted model without the interaction variable is only 0.804. Consequently, the F test for the significance of the interaction between gender and minority group status with respect to income is given as follows:

$$F = \frac{(R_{y.123}^2 - R_{y.12}^2)/(3-2)}{(1 - R_{y.123}^2)/(N-3-1)}$$

$$= \frac{(0.906 - 0.804)/1}{(1 - 0.906)/4} = \frac{0.102/1}{0.094/4}$$

$$= \frac{0.102}{0.024} = 4.25$$

In this particular example, the inclusion of an interaction variable increases the proportion of the variance in income explained by the model. However, the interaction between gender and minority group status is not statistically significant, due primarily to the extremely small sample size.

Finally, it must be noted that testing for interaction in analysis of variance using regression models with dummy variables can become fairly complicated whenever there are several categorical variables or whenever the categorical variables have several categories. For example, if we wish to test for interactions between gender and membership in either one of the two major minority groups with respect to income, we must construct two separate interaction variables. Specifically, if we wish to retain nonminority men as the excluded category, then we must construct one dummy interaction variable for African-American women and another for Hispanic-American women. However, once we have created these separate interaction variables, we can use the F test to test for the significance of all of these interaction variables at once. In particular, we can test the compound null hypothesis that the partial regression coefficients for all of these variables are equal to zero. Alternatively, we might have theoretical or substantive reasons to expect that only certain interaction variables are significant. For example, we might expect an interaction between gender and minority group status for African-American women but not for Hispanic-American women. In this case, we can use either the F test or the t test to determine whether or not the partial regression coefficient for a particular dummy interaction variable is significant.

CHAPTER 31

Analysis of Covariance
Using the Regression Model

Regression analysis typically involves the use of continuous independent variables to predict a continuous dependent variable. It is also possible, of course, to use categorical independent variables, in the form of dummy variables, to perform an analysis of variance using the regression model. It should come as no surprise, then, to learn that a regression model can include both continuous and categorical independent variables at the same time. This procedure is known as analysis of covariance. *Analysis of covariance is a multiple regression model that contains both continuous independent variables and categorical independent variables represented by dummy variables.* According to the conventions of analysis of covariance, the categorical variables are referred to as factors, whereas the continuous variables are referred to as covariates.

Analysis of covariance has many uses in social science research. To begin with, it can be used to assess the effect of one or more categorical variables on a dependent variable, controlling for the effects of one or more continuous variables. For example, we know that men have higher incomes on average than women. However, these differences between men and women with respect to income may be attributable, at least in part, to differences in their levels of education. In order to examine this explanation for the differences in income between men and women, we might assess the effect of gender on income, controlling for these differences in education. Specifically, we might conduct an analysis of covariance using a regression model that contains both a dummy independent variable for gender and a continuous independent variable for education. Specifically, let us consider a hypothetical example involving eight individuals: four men and four women. The regression model for this analysis of covariance, where y is the continuous dependent variable, income on thousands of dollars, x_1 is the dummy independent variable representing women, and x_2 is the continuous independent variable for education, measured in years of schooling, is given by:

$$\hat{y} = ua + x_1 b_{y1.2} + x_2 b_{y2.1} + e$$

where the vectors contain the following values:

$$
\begin{bmatrix} 21 \\ 27 \\ 23 \\ 25 \\ 19 \\ 21 \\ 17 \\ 15 \end{bmatrix}
=
\begin{bmatrix} 1 \\ 1 \\ 1 \\ 1 \\ 1 \\ 1 \\ 1 \\ 1 \end{bmatrix} a +
\begin{bmatrix} 0 \\ 0 \\ 0 \\ 0 \\ 1 \\ 1 \\ 1 \\ 1 \end{bmatrix} b_{y1.2} +
\begin{bmatrix} 12 \\ 16 \\ 13 \\ 13 \\ 15 \\ 16 \\ 12 \\ 12 \end{bmatrix} b_{y2.1} +
\begin{bmatrix} e_1 \\ e_2 \\ e_3 \\ e_4 \\ e_5 \\ e_6 \\ e_7 \\ e_8 \end{bmatrix}
$$

The application of ordinary least-squares estimation procedures to the multiple regression model for these data yields the following intercept and partial regression coefficients:

$$y = u(7.24) + x_1(-6.31) + x_2(1.24) + e$$

The parameters of this regression model tell us several things about the effects of gender and education on income. In any regression model, the intercept is equal to the expected value of the dependent variable whenever all of the independent variables are equal to zero. Therefore, in the case of an analysis of covariance model, the intercept represents the expected income for the observations in the excluded category whenever the covariate is equal to zero. In this particular case, the intercept of 7.32 tells us that the expected value of income for men with no education at all is $7,320. Similarly, in an analysis of covariance model, the partial regression coefficient for each dummy independent variable represents the expected difference on the dependent variable between that group and the group represented by the excluded category, controlling for the effects of other independent variables. The partial regression coefficient of –6.31 for the dummy variable representing women, x_1, tells us that women earn $6,310 less on average than men, controlling for the effects of education. Finally, in an analysis of covariance model, the partial regression coefficient for each continuous independent variable represents the expected change in the dependent variable associated with a one unit change in the independent variable, controlling for the effect of other independent variables. Therefore, the partial regression coefficient of 1.24 for the continuous education variable, x_2, tells us that each additional year of education yields an expected increment of $1,240 in income, controlling for the effects of gender.

Moreover, we can partition the variance in the dependent variable explained by each independent variable using the coefficient of semi-partial determination. However, since these two independent variables are not uncorrelated, the manner in which this variance is partitioned depends on the causal priority of the independent variables. In the case of the model assessing the effects of gender and education on income, it is reasonable to assume that gender is causally prior to education. Therefore, the variance in income explained by gender and education can be partitioned as follows:

$$R^2_{y(2.1)} = R^2_{y.12} - r^2_{y2}$$

$$= 0.942 - 0.643 = 0.299$$

In short, gender and education together explain 94.2 percent of the variance in income. However, gender alone explains 64.3 percent of the variance in income. Consequently, education explains 29.9 percent of the variance in income not already explained by gender.

It must be noted that the validity of these results depends on one important assumption: the homogeneity of regression. Simply stated, this assumption asserts that the relationship between the continuous independent variables and the dependent variable is the same for each category of the categorical independent variables. In other words, this model assumes that there is no interaction between the factors and the covariates. In order to test this assumption, it is necessary to construct variables that represent the interaction between the dummy variables representing the categorical independent variables and the continuous independent variables. In the case of the model assessing the effects of gender and education on income, it is necessary to create one inter-action variable that represents the interaction between the dummy variable representing women and the continuous education variable. This interaction variable is equal to the educations of the women only. The educations of the men are scored as zeros on this interaction vari-able. Once this interaction variable, x_3, has been created, it can be included in the regression model, along with the original independent variables, x_1 and x_2, as follows:

$$y = ua + x_1 b_{y1.23} + x_2 b_{y2.13} + x_3 b_{y3.12} + e$$

such that:

$$
\begin{bmatrix} 21 \\ 27 \\ 23 \\ 25 \\ 19 \\ 21 \\ 17 \\ 15 \end{bmatrix}
=
\begin{bmatrix} 1 \\ 1 \\ 1 \\ 1 \\ 1 \\ 1 \\ 1 \\ 1 \end{bmatrix} a
+
\begin{bmatrix} 0 \\ 0 \\ 0 \\ 0 \\ 1 \\ 1 \\ 1 \\ 1 \end{bmatrix} b_{y1.23}
+
\begin{bmatrix} 12 \\ 16 \\ 13 \\ 13 \\ 15 \\ 16 \\ 12 \\ 12 \end{bmatrix} b_{y2.13}
+
\begin{bmatrix} 0 \\ 0 \\ 0 \\ 0 \\ 15 \\ 16 \\ 12 \\ 12 \end{bmatrix} b_{y3.12}
+
\begin{bmatrix} e_1 \\ e_2 \\ e_3 \\ e_4 \\ e_5 \\ e_6 \\ e_7 \\ e_8 \end{bmatrix}
$$

The application of ordinary least-squares estimation procedures to the multiple regression model for these data yields the following intercept and partial regression coefficients:

$$y = u (6.00) + x_1 (-4.18) + x_2 (1.33) + x_3 (-0.16) + e$$

It can be seen that the regression coefficient for this interaction vari-able is relatively small in comparison to the regression coefficient for the education variable. Indeed, the coefficient of determination for this model with an interaction variable is 0.943. The t test for this partial regression coefficient indicates that this interaction variable is not statistically significant. Of course, the fact that this interaction variable is not statistically significant is attributable, in large part, to the extremely small sample size used in the example. This same hypothesis could have been tested using the F test to compare the coefficient of determination for a full model that contains the main effects variables and the interaction variable with the coefficient of determination for a restricted model that contains these same main effects variables but excludes the interaction variable. Indeed, whenever the categorical variable contains more than two categories, the F test must be used to assess the extent of interaction in the model as a whole.

It must be noted that, in many cases, we are not interested in the interactions between categorical and continuous independent variables with respect to a dependent variable. Indeed, the presence of statistically significant "interaction effects" complicates our interpretation of the "main effects" of the independent variables on a dependent variable. However, there are situations in which we have theoretical reasons to expect significant interactions between certain categorical independent variables and certain continuous independent variables with respect to a dependent variable. The interaction between gender and education with respect to income is an example of an interaction that has theoretical implications for understanding the income gap between men and women. In these situations, we must incorporate these interactions into our regression model. As we shall see, there are ways of incorporating interaction variables into regression models for analysis of covariance that render them more interpretable.

CHAPTER 32

Interpreting Interaction in Analysis of Covariance

It can be somewhat difficult to interpret the partial regression coefficients of a multiple regression model used to perform an analysis of covariance whenever this model includes interaction variables. This difficulty arises because the partial regression coefficient for an interaction variable represents the difference between the partial regression coefficients on a covariate for two groups. It may not be too difficult to interpret such a partial regression coefficient in a simple analysis of covariance model with only one dummy independent variable and one continuous independent variable, but the situation can become much more confusing in analysis of covariance models that contain more than one dummy independent variable or more than one continuous independent variable. Fortunately, there is an alternative procedure for assessing the effect of interaction in analysis of covariance models that yields partial regression coefficients that are much easier to interpret.

In order to demonstrate this procedure, let us consider once again the regression model used to perform an analysis of covariance of the effects of gender and education on income. As before, the categorical gender variable is incorporated into the model using a dummy variable, x_1, that represents women. This implies, of course, that men are the excluded category in this analysis. Education is incorporated into the model by a continuous variable, x_2, representing the number of years of schooling. Moreover, this model also contains an interaction variable, x_3, representing the interaction of gender and education with respect to income. This interaction variable is equal to the educations of the women only; the educations of the men are equal to zero. As noted earlier, the parameters of the multiple regression model for this analysis of covariance with interaction yields the following intercept and partial regression coefficients:

$$y = u\,(6.00) + x_1\,(-4.18) + x_2\,(1.33) + x_3\,(-0.16) + e$$

The parameters of this model are easily interpreted, if we consider the fact that this model, in effect, incorporates separate prediction equations for men and women. Specifically, the prediction equation for the men in this sample is given by:

$$\hat{y}_m = u\,(6.00) + x_2\,(1.33)$$

This equation for the predicted incomes of men does not include the dummy variable for the effect of being a woman or the interaction variable representing the effect of education for women. This equation clearly demonstrates that the partial regression coefficient for the continuous education variable, x_2, represents the effect of education on income for men. Similarly, the prediction equation for the women in this sample is given by:

$$\hat{y}_w = u\,(6.00) + x_1\,(-4.18) + x_2\,(1.33) + x_3\,(-0.16)$$

This equation for the predicted incomes of women includes all of the variables contained in the prediction equation for men, but it also includes the dummy variable for the effect of being a women and the interaction variable representing the difference in the effect of education for women relative to men. This last prediction equation suggests that the effect of education on income for women is equal to the sum of the partial regression coefficient for the effect of education on income for men, $b_{y2.13}$, and the difference in the effect of education on income for women relative to men, $b_{y3.12}$, as follows:

$$b_{y2.13} + b_{y3.12} = 1.33 - 0.16$$

$$= 1.17$$

In short, men can expect an increase of $1,330 in income for every additional year of education, whereas women can expect an increase of only $1,170 in income for every additional year of education.

It is important to note that we can obtain the same estimates of the separate effects of education on income for men and women using a multiple regression model for analysis of covariance with interaction that contains separate interaction variables for the interaction of education and gender. Specifically, we can delete the continuous variable for education and include an interaction variable for the effect of education for men, x_4, as follows:

$$y = ua + x_1 b_{y1.34} + x_3 b_{y3.14} + x_4 b_{y4.13} + e$$

such that:

$$
\begin{bmatrix} 21 \\ 27 \\ 23 \\ 25 \\ 19 \\ 21 \\ 17 \\ 15 \end{bmatrix}
=
\begin{bmatrix} 1 \\ 1 \\ 1 \\ 1 \\ 1 \\ 1 \\ 1 \\ 1 \end{bmatrix} a +
\begin{bmatrix} 0 \\ 0 \\ 0 \\ 0 \\ 1 \\ 1 \\ 1 \\ 1 \end{bmatrix} b_{y1.34} +
\begin{bmatrix} 0 \\ 0 \\ 0 \\ 0 \\ 15 \\ 16 \\ 12 \\ 12 \end{bmatrix} b_{y3.14} +
\begin{bmatrix} 12 \\ 16 \\ 13 \\ 13 \\ 0 \\ 0 \\ 0 \\ 0 \end{bmatrix} b_{y4.13} +
\begin{bmatrix} e_1 \\ e_2 \\ e_3 \\ e_4 \\ e_5 \\ e_6 \\ e_7 \\ e_8 \end{bmatrix}
$$

The application of ordinary least-squares estimation procedures to the multiple regression model for these data yields the following intercept and partial regression coefficients:

$$y = u\,(6.00) + x_1\,(-4.18) + x_3\,(1.17) + x_4\,(1.33) + e$$

Not surprisingly, this regression model gives us results that are consistent with the previous regression model. The intercept and the partial regression coefficients for the dummy variable representing women are the same in both models. Moreover, the partial regression coefficients for the effect of education in income for men are the same, although the interpretation of this coefficient in the second model is less ambiguous. The only difference between the two models is that the partial regression coefficient, $b_{y4.13}$, in the second model is directly interpretable as the effect of education on income for women. Of course, the coefficients of determination for these two models are also identical. These similarities should not surprise us because these two models contain exactly the same information. These models differ only in the manner in which this information is incorporated in the model. The advantage of incorporating separate variables representing the interaction between a continuous independent variable and a categorical independent variable into a regression model whenever there are significant interaction effects is that the interpretation of the partial regression coefficients in terms of interaction effects is straightforward and unambiguous. Moreover, this procedure can readily be extended to much larger and more complicated models.

CHAPTER 33

Structural Equation Models and Path Analysis

In multiple regression analysis, we are normally concerned with the relationship between a single dependent variable and two or more independent variables. We recognize that these independent variables may be correlated with one another, but we are not always interested in the relationships among them. There are times, however, when we wish to examine the relationships among the independent variables in our analysis. In these instances, we must estimate the parameters of more than one regression equation because we are interested in a model that contains more than a single dependent variable. Indeed, we are interested in a model in which a dependent variable in one regression equation is an independent variable in another regression equation. *Multiple equation models in which a dependent variable in one equation appears as an independent variable in another equation are referred to as structural equation models.*

In order to understand the logic of structural equation models, let us consider the simplest possible structural equation model, one with three variables and two equations. The theory of status attainment asserts that income is determined by educational and occupational achievement. This theory also asserts that occupational achievement is determined by educational achievement. We can write the regression equations corresponding to these two theoretical statements as follows:

$$x_2 \ = \ ua \ + \ x_3 b_{23} \ + \ e_2$$

$$x_1 \ = \ ua \ + \ x_3 b_{13.2} \ + \ x_2 b_{12.3} \ + \ e_1$$

where variable x_1 is individual income, measured in thousands of dollars, variable x_2 is individual occupational achievement, measured on a scale of occupational prestige, and variable x_3 is individual educational achievement, measured in years of schooling.

This is a very simple structural equation model. One of the most important statistical properties of this particular model is that the dependent variables do not have any effects on any of the independent variables that affect them. For instance, income, x_1, has no effect on either occupation, x_2, or education, x_3. Similarly, occupation, x_2, has no effect on education, x_3. In short, this structural equation model does not permit any reciprocal causation. *A structural equation model that does not contain reciprocal causation is known as a recursive model.* One advantage of recursive models is that we can obtain unbiased estimates of the parameters of the structural equation model using ordinary least-squares estimation procedures. Indeed, the parameters of this model are equivalent to the corresponding simple or partial regression coefficients obtained from these regression equations.

One technique for analyzing a structural equation model is path analysis. *Path analysis involves the use of structural equation models with standardized variables.* One of the primary purposes of path analysis is to reveal the relative effects of each variable on other variables in the model. In order to facilitate these comparisons, all of the variables are expressed as standardized variables with zero means and unit variances. In practice, this means that we focus on the standardized regression coefficients rather than the corresponding unstandardized regression coefficients. In path analysis, standardized partial regression coefficients are referred to as path coefficients. As such, they represent the causal effect of one variable on another, controlling for the causal effects of other variables. Because they are nothing more than standardized regression coefficients, these path coefficients measure causal effects in terms of the expected standard deviation change in the dependent variable produced by a one standard deviation change in the independent variable, holding constant any other independent variables.

In order to see the utility of this technique, let us consider once again the simple structural equation model of the relationship between income, education, and occupation. We can express this structural equation model as a path analysis model by simply replacing the unstandardized variables with the corresponding standardized variables as follows:

$$z_2 = z_3 b_{23}^* + e_2$$

$$z_1 = z_3 b_{13.2}^* + z_2 b_{12.3}^* + e_1$$

where the asterisks indicate that the regression coefficients are standardized regression coefficients. It will be noted that there are no intercepts in the path equations because the intercept is equal to zero whenever all of the variables in an equation have been expressed as deviation from their means, as is the case with standardized variables.

Using sample data on the income, education, and occupation of men, the least-squares estimates of the standardized partial regression coefficients are given as follows:

$$z_2 = z_3 (0.643) + e_2$$

$$z_1 = z_3 (0.157) + z_2 (0.341) + e_1$$

These path coefficients tell us a great deal about the relative effects of education and occupation on income. For example, the path coefficient in the first equation tells us that a one standard deviation change in education, x_3, produces a 0.643 standard deviation change in occupation, x_2. Similarly, the first path coefficient in the second equation tells us that a one standard deviation change in education, x_3, controlling for occupation, x_2, produces only a 0.157 standard deviation change in income, x_1. However, the second path coefficient in the second equation tells us that a one standard deviation change in occupation, x_2, controlling for education, x_3, produces a 0.341 standard deviation change in income, x_1. Within the context of this model, these results indicate that the direct effect of occupation on income, controlling for education, is twice as large as the direct effect of education on income, controlling for occupation. At the same time, we cannot conclude that education is not an important variable in the model because, even though it has only a modest direct effect on income, it does have a very substantial direct effect on occupation.

Path analysis is especially useful in examining relatively large causal models in which a variable can affect other variables through multiple paths. In order to evaluate the utility of this technique, let us consider a slightly more complicated model. Specifically, let us add father's education, x_4, to the model explaining the incomes of men in terms of their education and occupation. The path diagram that

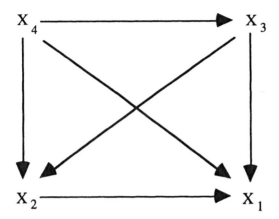

Figure 33.1. Path Diagram of Status Attainment Model

specifies the relationships between these variables is presented in Figure 33.1. Each arrow signifies a direct causal effect between two variables. To begin with, this diagram indicates that father's education, x_4, has direct effects on son's education, x_3, son's occupation, x_2, and son's income, x_1. Similarly, son's education, x_3, has direct effects on son's occupation, x_2, and son's income, x_1. Finally, son's occupation, x_2, has direct effects on son's income, x_1.

The path coefficients for this model are given by the standardized partial regression coefficients for the following equations:

$$z_3 = z_4 b_{34}^* + e_3$$

$$z_2 = z_4 b_{24.3}^* + z_3 b_{23.4}^* + e_2$$

$$z_1 = z_4 b_{14.23}^* + z_3 b_{13.24}^* + z_2 b_{12.34}^* + z_1$$

where variable z_4 represents father's education, variable z_3 represents son's education, variable z_2 represents son's occupation, and variable z_1 represents son's income.

Using sample data on income, education, occupation, and father's education for men, the least-squares estimates of the standardized regression coefficients, or path coefficients, are given as follows:

$$z_3 = z_4 (0.405) + e_3$$

$$z_2 = z_4 (0.071) + z_3 (0.614) + e_2$$

$$z_1 = z_4 (0.073) + z_3 (0.132) + z_2 (0.334) + e_1$$

It can be seen that the inclusion of father's education into this path model does not alter much the basic results obtained for the earlier model. The path coefficients for the effects of both son's education and occupation on son's income and the path coefficient for the effect of son's education on son's occupation are relatively unchanged. However, the path coefficients for this model tell us a great deal about the effects of father's education on all of these variables. For example, a one standard deviation change in father's education, x_4, produces only a 0.073 standard deviation change in son's income, x_1, and only a 0.071 standard deviation change in son's occupation, x_2, but it does produce a 0.405 standard deviation change in the son's education, x_3. In short, father's education has a substantial direct effect on son's education but only negligible direct effects on son's occupation or income.

Structural equation models are extremely useful for examining the relationships among a set of variables. Specifically, these models enable us to trace out the direct effects of one variable on another as well as the indirect effects of one variable on another that are transmitted through other variables. Path analysis simplifies this process by requiring that all of the variables be expressed in standard form. In this way, it is possible to compare the effects of different variables. In the case of the status attainment model, for example, path analysis reveals that education affects income primarily through occupation. It also reveals that any effect of father's education on this process is transmitted primarily through son's education. It is worth noting that the results obtained from structural equation models such as path analysis are a product of the particular theoretical structure that we imposed on the data. Of course, different theoretical specifications of the structural equation model describing the relationships within a set of variables invariably yield different empirical results.

CHAPTER 34

Computing Direct and Total Effects of Variables

One of the lessons to be drawn from structural equation models and path analysis is that an independent variable can have both direct and indirect effects on a dependent variable. In other words, some of the effects of an independent variable on a dependent variable may be transmitted through intervening variables. Consequently, the partial regression coefficient for an independent variable in a multiple regression equation may not capture all of its effects on the dependent variable. In order to understand the difference between direct and total effects, let us consider the example of the simple structural equation model that explains income in terms of education and occupation. The relationship between these three variables was represented by the following set of structural equations, where the variables are expressed in standard form:

$$z_2 = z_3 b_{23}^* + e_2$$

$$z_1 = z_3 b_{13.2}^* + z_2 b_{12.3}^* + e_1$$

where variable z_3 is education, variable z_2 is occupation, and variable z_1 is education. It is evident from these structural equations that a one unit change in variable z_3 will produce a change in variable z_2 and a change in variable z_3. In turn, the change in variable z_2 produced by a change in variable z_3 will produce a further change in variable z_1.

Given this structural equation model of the relationship between education, occupation, and income, it is apparent that education has a direct effect on income that is independent of occupation as well as an indirect effect that is transmitted through occupation. Therefore, the total effect of education on income is the sum of its direct effect and its indirect effect transmitted through occupation. The direct effect of education on income, d_{13}, is given by the corresponding standardized partial regression coefficient as follows:

$$d_{13} = b^*_{13.2}$$

However, in order to compute the total effect of education on income, we must substitute the structural equation for occupation into the structural equation for income. Therefore, the total effect of education on income, t_{13}, is given by the sum of its direct and indirect effects as follows:

$$t_{13} = d_{13} + (d_{23}d_{12})$$

$$= b^*_{13.2} + (b^*_{23} \, b^*_{12.3})$$

The last term on the right, which represents the indirect effects of education on income, is simply the product of the direct effect of education, x_3, on occupation, x_2, and its direct effect on income, x_1.

In order to calculate the direct and total effects of education on income, it is necessary to use the path coefficients associated with this structural equation model given by:

$$z_2 = z_1 (0.643) + e_2$$

$$z_1 = z_3 (0.157) + z_2 (0.341) + e_1$$

Using these path coefficients, the direct and total effects of education on income can be computed as follows:

$$d_{13} = b^*_{13.2} = 0.157$$

$$t_{13} = b^*_{13.2} + (b^*_{23} \, b^*_{12.3}) = 0.157 + (0.643)(0.341)$$

$$= 0.157 + 0.219 = 0.376$$

In short, a one standard deviation change in income will produce a 0.376 standard deviation change in income. However, most of the total effect of education is transmitted indirectly through the intervening occupation variable.

The decomposition of the total effect of a variable on another variable into direct and indirect effects can become very complicated in the case of elaborate path models. In order to examine this problem, let us consider the more complicated path model that explains son's income in terms of father's education as well as son's education and occupation. The structural equations for this model are given by:

$$z_3 = z_4 b_{34}^* + e_3$$

$$z_2 = z_4 b_{24.3}^* + z_3 b_{23.4}^* + e_2$$

$$z_1 = z_4 b_{14.23}^* + z_3 b_{13.24}^* + z_2 b_{12.34}^* + e_1$$

where variable z_4 is father's education, variable z_3 is son's education, variable z_2 is son's occupation, and variable z_1 is son's income.

The equation for the total effect of father's education on son's income can be obtained by substituting the first equation into the second equation and then substituting the second equation into the third equation. In this way, it is possible to calculate the total effect of a unit change in father's education on son's income. Specifically, these calculations reveal that father's education has indirect effects on son's income through three different paths. Consequently, the total effect of father's education on son's income, t_{14}, is given by:

$$t_{14} = d_{14} + (d_{34}d_{13}) + (d_{24}d_{12}) + (d_{34}d_{23}d_{12})$$

$$= b_{14.23}^* + (b_{34}^* b_{13.24}^*) + (b_{24.3}^* b_{12.34}^*) + (b_{34}^* b_{23.4}^* b_{12.34}^*)$$

The first term on the right is, of course, the direct effect of father's education, z_4, on income, z_1. The second term is the indirect effect of father's education, z_4, on income, z_1, transmitted through son's education, z_3. The third term is the indirect effect of father's education, z_4, on income, z_1, transmitted through son's occupation, z_2. Finally, the last term is the indirect effect of father's education, z_4, on son's income, z_1, transmitted through education, z_3, and then through occupation, z_2.

In order to calculate the direct and total effects of father's education on son's income, it is necessary to use the path coefficients associated with this structural equation model given by:

$$z_3 = z_4 (0.405) + e_3$$

$$z_2 = z_4 (0.071) + z_3 (0.614) + e_2$$

$$z_1 = z_4 (0.073) + z_3 (0.132) + z_2 (0.334) + z_1$$

Given these path coefficients, the total effect of father's education on son's income can be computed as follows:

$$t_{14} = 0.073 + (0.405)(0.132) + (0.071)(0.334)$$

$$+ (0.405)(0.614)(0.334)$$

$$= 0.073 + 0.053 + 0.024 + 0.083$$

$$= 0.233$$

In this case, it is apparent that the total effects of father's education on son's income far exceed its direct effects. In short, most of the effects of father's education on son's income is transmitted through son's education and occupation.

As this relatively simple example demonstrates, the calculations required to estimate the total effects of one variable on another can be quite laborious. Fortunately, it is possible to circumvent these onerous calculations. Specifically, it can be demonstrated that the total effect of an independent variable on a dependent variable is equal to its regression coefficient in a regression equation for that dependent variable that includes any causally prior variables but excludes any intervening variables. *In other words, the total effect of a variable is its effect on a dependent variable, controlling for the effects of causally prior variables but ignoring the effects of intervening variables.* However, if the independent variable in question is an exogenous variable, one that is not a dependent variable in any of the structural equations, then it is necessary to control for the effects of any other exogenous variables as well. This result can be verified by noting that the simple regression coefficient between son's education,

z_3, and income, z_1, in the first structural equation model with just three variables is equal to the total effect of education on income such that:

$$b_{13}^* = 0.376 = t_{13}$$

Similarly, the simple regression coefficient between father's education, z_4, and son's income, z_1, in the second structural equation model with four variables is equal the total effect of father's education on son's income such that:

$$b_{14}^* = 0.233 = t_{14}$$

Conversely, the direct effect of any variable is equal to its simple or partial regression coefficient, controlling for both causally prior variables and intervening variables. *In other words, the direct effect of a variable is its effect on a dependent variable, controlling for the effects of both causally prior and intervening variables.* Once again, if the independent variable is an exogenous variable, then it is necessary to control for the effects of any other exogenous variables as well. Of course, if there are no intervening variables between an independent variable and the dependent variable, then the direct effect of a variable is equal to its total effect.

Using this procedure, it is possible to compute the direct and total effects of any independent variable in a structural equation model on any other dependent variable in that model. Indeed, it is sometimes useful to compare the total and direct effects of one or more independent variables on a dependent variable even if we are not interested in all of the parameters of the fully specified structural equation model. In particular, it is often sufficient to differentiate simply between the exogenous variables and the endogenous variables in an analysis and to compare the total effects of the exogenous variables with their direct effects. For example, we might compare the total effects of several exogenous family background variables, such as father's education and occupation, on son's income with their direct effects, once the endogenous individual achievement variables, such as son's education and occupation, have been incorporated into the model. A regression equation that includes only the exogenous variables that affect a dependent variable is often referred to as the "reduced form equation."

CHAPTER 35

Model Specification
in Regression Analysis

One of the most important but least understood issues in all of regression analysis concerns model specification. *Model specification refers to the determination of which independent variables should be included in or excluded from a regression equation.* In general, the specification of a regression model should be based primarily on theoretical considerations rather than empirical or methodological ones. A multiple regression model is, in fact, a theoretical statement about the causal relationship between one or more independent variables and a dependent variable. Indeed, it can be observed that regression analysis involves three distinct stages: the specification of a model, the estimation of the parameters of this model, and the interpretation of these parameters. Specification is the first and most critical of these stages. Our estimates of the parameters of a model and our interpretation of them depend on the correct specification of the model. Consequently, problems can arise whenever we misspecify a model. There are two basic types of specification errors. In the first, we misspecify a model by including in the regression equation an independent variable that is theoretically irrelevant. In the second, we misspecify the model by excluding from the regression equation an independent variable that is theoretically relevant. Both types of specification errors can lead to problems of estimation and interpretation.

   It must be noted, at the outset, that specification errors are not especially problematic whenever the independent variables in a multiple regression model are orthogonal or uncorrelated with one another. It will be recalled that the partial regression coefficients for a set of orthogonal independent variables in a multiple regression equation are equal to their respective simple regression coefficients. Consequently, the addition or deletion of an orthogonal independent variable does not have any effect on the partial regression coefficients of the other independent variables in the regression equation. However, the addition or deletion of an orthogonal independent variable will affect the standard errors of the partial regression coefficients of other independent variables in the equation. Specifically, the addition of an independent variable to a regression equation will increase the standard errors of the partial regression coefficients by decreasing their degrees of freedom. At the same time, however, the addition of an independent variable to a regression equation may decrease these same standard errors by decreasing the error variance in the dependent variable. Conversely, the deletion of an independent variable from a regression equation will decrease the standard errors of the partial regression coefficients by increasing their degrees of freedom. However, once again, the deletion of an independent variable may increase the standard errors of the partial regression coefficients by decreasing the error variance of the dependent variable.

Of course, orthogonal independent variables are a rarity. In practice, the independent variables in a multiple regression equation are often correlated with one another to some extent. Unfortunately, specification errors are more problematic in models that contain correlated independent variables because the partial regression coefficient of each independent variable is likely to be affected by the inclusion or exclusion of other independent variables. We can demonstrate the problems association with specification errors using a familiar example. This example involves the regression of income on education and occupation. Specifically, the multiple regression of income on these two independent variables, in the case of standardized variables, is given by:

$$z_1 = z_2 (0.341) + z_3 (0.157) + e$$

where variable z_1 is income, variable z_2 is occupation, and variable z_3 is education. In this particular case, we have employed standardized variables because they allow us to compare directly the partial regression coefficients of the different independent variables. We shall assume that this model is correctly specified inasmuch as it contains the theoretically relevant predictors of income.

Next, we can consider the situation in which we have included in a regression equation a theoretically irrelevant independent variable that is correlated with the other independent variables in that equation. In this situation, we are likely to obtain different estimates of the partial regression coefficients of those independent variables. Moreover, the magnitude of the change in these partial regression coefficients is determined by the degree of correlation among these independent variables. We can demonstrate the effect of including an irrelevant independent variable on the partial regression coefficients of the other independent variables in a regression equation using this same empirical example. Specifically, we can introduce a specification error by including an irrelevant independent variable, father's education, to this regression equation. The multiple regression of income on these three independent variables, in the case of standardized variables, is given by:

$$z_1 = z_2 (0.334) + z_3 (0.132) + z_4 (0.073) + e$$

where variable z_1 is individual income, variable z_2 is individual occupational prestige, variable z_3 is individual education, and variable z_4 is father's education. We shall assume that this model is incorrectly specified because we have no theoretical rationale for expecting that father's education has any direct effect on son's income. In this particular case, the addition of this irrelevant independent variable to this regression equation has a relatively negligible effect on the partial regression coefficients of the other independent variables. The relatively negligible effect that the inclusion of this irrelevant independent variable has on the partial regression coefficients of the other independent variables is probably due to the fact that it is not highly correlated with the dependent variable.

Finally, we can consider the opposite situation in which we have excluded from a regression equation a theoretically relevant independent variable that is correlated with the other independent variables in that equation. In this situation, we are likely to obtain different estimates of the partial regression coefficients of those independent variables. Once again, the change in these partial regression coefficients is directly related to the extent to which the excluded independent variable is correlated with the independent variables in this equation. We can demonstrate the effect of excluding a relevant independent variable on the partial regression coefficients of the other independent variables in a regression equation using the same example.

Specifically, we can introduce a specification error by excluding occupation, z_2, from this regression equation. The simple regression of income on education, in the case of standardized variables, is given by:

$$z_1 = z_3 (0.376) + e$$

where variable z_1 is income and variable z_3 is education. It is evident that the standardized simple regression coefficient for the regression of income on education is much larger than the standardized partial regression coefficient for the regression of income on education, controlling for occupation. In this situation, we might be led to over-estimate the effects of education on income.

In general, the problems associated with the exclusion of a theoretically relevant independent variable from a regression equation are more serious than the problems associated with the inclusion of a theoretically irrelevant independent variable. Whenever we exclude a relevant independent variable from a regression model, we are likely to ignore the fact that its effects are probably being captured, at least in part, by those independent variables that we have included in the model. Conversely, whenever we include an irrelevant independent variable to a regression model, we are more likely to be aware of the fact that it is probably capturing some of the effects of the other independent variables in the model. Consequently, we must be careful about excluding independent variables from our models, even when they are not statistically significant. Indeed, an independent variable may fail to achieve statistical significance merely because it is highly correlated with the other independent variables. In this regard, it might be noted that there is an intimate relationship between the problem of specification error and the problem of multicollinearity.

These results suggest that we must always be aware of the possible effects of specification error on our results. In practice, the problem of specification error is often complicated by the fact that we may be working with relatively "weak" theories. For a variety of reasons, we are not always able to draw upon a well developed and highly coherent theory in specifying our regression models. Consequently, there is sometimes considerable theoretical ambiguity as to the relevance of particular independent variables. In these situations, we should be prepared to present the results of alternative specifications of our model. In this way, we are able to examine the effects of including

Table 35.1. Alternative Regression Models of the Income
Attainment Process

Independent variables	Model 1	Model 2	Model 3
Occupation (z_2)	0.341	0.334	
Education (z_3)	0.157	0.132	0.376
Father's education (z_4)		0.073	
R^2	0.141	0.214	0.210

potentially irrelevant independent variables in a model as well as the
effects of excluding potentially relevant independent variables. For
example, three alternative specifications of the income attainment
model are presented in Table 35.1. By presenting the parameter estimates associated with alternative models in this manner, we are able to
compare the effects of different specifications of the model both in
terms of the partial regression coefficients associated with particular
variables and in terms of the coefficient of determination associated
with each specification of the model.

CHAPTER 36

Influential Cases in
Regression Analysis

In regression analysis, we must be aware of the fact that our results may be affected by the presence of a few influential cases. Due to the very nature of ordinary least-squares estimation procedures, not all of the cases in an analysis are equal in terms of their ability to influence the parameters of the regression equation. The basic problem with influential cases is that they have an inordinate impact on the results of our regression analysis. Consequently, we might have obtained somewhat different results if these influential cases had not been included in our analysis. Indeed, the best definition of an influential case, both statistically and intuitively, relies on this property. *An influential case is any case that significantly alters the value of a regression coefficient whenever it is deleted from an analysis.* If the deletion of particular cases in an analysis alters the parameters of the regression equation significantly, then these cases represent influential cases. In general, influential cases have relatively extreme values on the independent variable and somewhat discrepant values on the dependent variable. In this context, the value of the dependent variable for a particular case can be viewed as discrepant to the extent that it deviates from its predicted value based on a regression equation derived from all of the other cases.

In order to demonstrate the problem of influential cases, let us consider a hypothetical example, involving seven observations, of the simple regression of a dependent variable, y, on an independent variable, x. The plot of these seven cases is presented in Figure 36.1. In

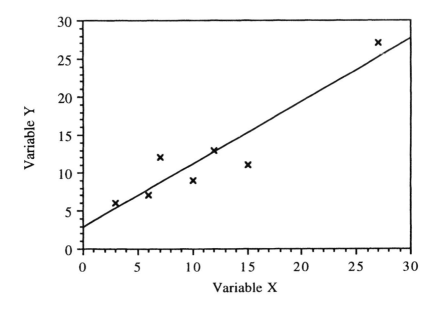

Figure 36.1. Regression with Influential Case

this particular example, which involves a simple regression between two variables, we can identify the potential influential case from a visual inspection of the plot of these seven cases on the dependent and the independent variables. One of the cases clearly has an extreme value on variable x and a slightly discrepant value on variable y. Given this fact, we might suspect that this case exerts an inordinate influence on the value of the regression coefficient.

Although it is often possible to identify potential influential cases from a visual inspection of the plot between a dependent variable and a single independent variable, it is much more difficult to identify influential cases in this manner in multiple regression models that include several independent variables. An alternative procedure for identifying influential cases, which applies to multiple regression models as well as simple regression models, involves the successive deletion of individual cases from the analysis. We can illustrate this procedure using this simple example. The least-squares estimates of

Table 36.1. Simple Regression of Y on X with One Case Deleted

Case deleted	Y	X	Regression coefficient	Change in coefficient
1	6	3	0.855	−0.027
2	7	6	0.816	0.012
3	12	7	0.879	−0.051
4	9	10	0.819	0.009
5	13	12	0.827	0.001
6	11	15	0.875	−0.047
7	27	27	0.450	0.378

the parameters of the simple regression equation for all seven hypothetical cases is given by:

$$y = u \ (2.685) + x \ (0.828) + e$$

Since the intercept of the regression equation is a simple function of the regression coefficient and the means of the variables, we are primarily interested in how the addition or deletion of a particular observation affects the regression coefficient. Table 36.1 presents the regression coefficients associated with seven separate regression analyses, each excluding one of the seven cases. The last column of this table shows the difference between the regression coefficient for the analysis including all seven case and the regression coefficient for the analysis that excludes a particular case. As this table reveals, the case with the most extreme value on variable x is the most influential case. The exclusion of this case from our analysis changes our results dramatically. The plot of the six remaining cases and their simple regression equation are presented in Figure 36.2. The least-squares

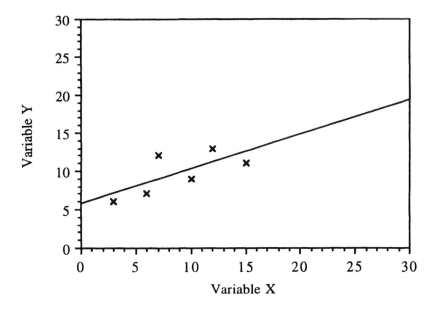

Figure 36.2. Regression without Influential Case

estimates of the parameters of this simple regression equation, with the influential case excluded from the analysis, are given by:

$$y = u\,(5.692) + x\,(0.450) + e$$

It is apparent that regression coefficient is smaller as a result of the deletion of the one influential case.

Although deleting cases from an analysis is the most certain method for identifying influential cases and their exact influence on the results of a regression analysis, this procedure is unwieldy in the case of large samples. For that reason, statisticians have developed a series of influence measures that can be very useful in identifying influential cases. A number of different influence measures have been proposed, but most of them are related to one another. These

Table 36.2.   Leverage, Discrepancy, and Cook's D Values for All Cases in Simple Regression of Y on X

Case	Leverage	Discrepancy	Cook's D
1	0.331	0.334	0.034
2	0.221	−0.240	0.010
3	0.195	1.644	0.244
4	0.148	−0.732	0.051
5	0.144	0.135	0.002
6	0.177	−2.141	0.286
7	0.785	1.894	4.310

influence measures generally focus on either the "leverage" or the "discrepancy" of each case. Three different influence measures for all seven cases in our hypothetical example are presented in Table 36.2. The leverage measure is a function of the value of the independent variable and its relationship to the other independent variables. As such, it measures the contribution of each case to the predicted value of the dependent variable. These particular leverage values are known as "hat values." The discrepancy measure is a function of the error of prediction associated with each case. These particular discrepancy values are known as "studentized residuals." Finally, the measure referred to as "Cook's D" is a multiplicative function of both the leverage and the discrepancy of each case. As this example suggests, a case is influential, according to Cook's D, whenever it possesses both a high level of leverage and a high level of discrepancy.

CHAPTER 37

The Problem of Multicollinearity

It will be recalled that one of the factors that affects the standard error of a partial regression coefficient is the degree to which that independent variable is correlated with the other independent variables in the regression equation. Other things being equal, an independent variable that is very highly correlated with one or more other independent variables will have a relatively large standard error. This implies that the partial regression coefficient is unstable and will vary greatly from one sample to the next. This is the situation known as multicollinearity. *Multicollinearity exists whenever an independent variable is highly correlated with one or more of the other independent variables in a multiple regression equation.* Multicollinearity is a problem because it undermines the statistical significance of an independent variable. Other things being equal, the larger the standard error of a regression coefficient, the less likely it is that this coefficient will be statistically significant.

Multicollinearity is one of the most vexing and intractable problems in all of regression analysis. Before examining this problem, we must distinguish between extreme multicollinearity and perfect multicollinearity. Perfect multicollinearity obtains whenever one independent variable is a perfect linear function of one or more of the other independent variables in a regression equation. This situation usually occurs whenever we construct a variable as a linear function of other variables. For example, we might construct a composite measure that is a simple additive function of several variables. A problem will arise, however, if we include this composite measure and the variables used to construct it as independent variables in the same regression equation. Ordinary least-squares estimation procedures will fail in this situation because all of the variance in the composite measure can be explained by the variables used to construct it. In mathematical terms, it will not be possible to calculate the inverse of the matrix of the covariances among the independent variables. This problem can also arise in dummy variable regression analysis whenever we fail to exclude one of the categories of a categorical variable from the analysis. If we include binary variables for all of the categories of a categorical variable in the regression equation, the intercept will be a simple additive function of these binary variables. Once again, ordinary least-squares estimation procedures will fail

Even less than perfect multicollinearity is a problem in regression analysis. Indeed, extreme multicollinearity is often a more difficult problem because it frequently goes undetected. Extreme multicollinearity occurs whenever an independent variable is very highly correlated with one or more other independent variables. In this situation, the partial regression coefficient for the independent variable in question will have a comparatively large standard error. In practice, multicollinearity often takes the form of two very highly correlated independent variables. Whenever two independent variables are very highly correlated with one another, neither or them is likely to be statistically significant, even though they may both be highly correlated with the dependent variable. The partial regression coefficients for both of these independent variables will have relatively large standard errors precisely because they are highly correlated with one another. Indeed, we can often detect the presence of extreme multicollinearity in a multiple regression equation by simply examining the magnitude of the standard errors of the partial regression coefficients. It will be recalled that a regression coefficient must be larger than its standard error in order to be statistically significant. Indeed, at the conventional 5 percent probability level, a regression coefficient must be almost twice as large as its standard error. Therefore, whenever we find a partial regression coefficient whose standard error is relatively large, we must consider the possibility of multicollinearity.

If we suspect that an independent variable in a regression equation suffers from multicollinearity, it is necessary to identify the source of the problem. We can sometimes identify pairs of highly correlated independent variables by inspecting the matrix of correlations among the independent variables. However, this procedure will only identify multicollinearity produced by the correlation between pairs of independent variables. It is possible for an independent variable to be highly correlated with several other independent variables without being highly correlated with any one of them. In order to examine this possibility, we must inspect the coefficients of determination between each independent variable and all of the other independent variables in a regression equation. If the computer programs used to perform the multiple regression analysis can provide the inverse of the matrix of the correlations among the independent variable, it is possible to obtain these coefficients of determination using the main diagonal elements of this inverse matrix. Specifically, each coefficient of determination is given by:

$$R^2_{i.jk} = 1 - \left(\frac{1}{r^{ii}} \right)$$

where r^{ii} is the diagonal element in row and column i of this inverse matrix. In any event, this procedure allows us to identify which independent variables are highly correlated with the other independent variables in the regression equation.

Although multicollinearity is a relatively easy problem to detect, it is not an easy problem to resolve. Indeed, several different statistical procedures have been devised for dealing with this problem. The most popular of these procedures is known as "ridge regression." In this procedure, the matrix of covariances among the independent variables is modified slightly in order to reduce the standard errors of the partial regression coefficients. Specifically, a relatively small positive value is added to the variance of each independent variable prior to calculating the least-squares estimates of the partial regression coefficients as follows :

$$\tilde{B} = \tilde{C}^{-1}_{xx} c_{yx} = (X'X + Ik)^{-1} X'y$$

such that

$$\tilde{C}^{-1} = \begin{bmatrix} s_1^2 + k & c_{12} & \cdots & c_{1j} \\ c_{21} & s_2^2 + k & \cdots & c_{2j} \\ \vdots & \vdots & & \vdots \\ c_{j1} & c_{j2} & \cdots & s_j^2 + k \end{bmatrix}$$

where k is the ridge regression constant that is added to the variance of each independent variable.

These ridge regression estimates of the partial regression coefficients will have smaller standard errors than their ordinary least-squares counterparts. However, the ridge regression estimates of the partial regression coefficients will also be biased. In short, ridge regression overcomes the problem of extreme multicollinearity by introducing a small amount of bias into the partial regression coefficients in order to reduce their standard errors. In practice, the main difficulty in using ridge regression involves the selection of an appropriate ridge regression constant to add to the main diagonal of the matrix of covariances among the independent variables. The objective is to find a constant that substantially reduces the standard errors of the partial regression coefficients without greatly increasing the bias of those coefficients. We can assess the degree of bias introduced into the partial regression coefficients associated with various ridge regression estimates by comparing them to the ordinary least-squares estimates of those same partial regression coefficients. After all, despite the fact that they have large standard errors in the presence of extreme multicollinearity, ordinary least-squares estimates of the partial regression coefficients are unbiased.

Obviously, ridge regression provides a less than ideal solution to the problem of multicollinearity. In fact, the simplest and most common solution to this problem is to avoid it altogether by respecifying the multiple regression equation. For example, we can often circumvent the problem of multicollinearity by deleting an independent variable from the analysis. This solution to the problem is most appropriate whenever multicollinearity is the result of two highly correlated independent variables. In this case, the deletion of one of the two variables from the analysis can often be justified on the grounds that these variables are simply redundant measures of the same underlying theoretical construct. In this regard, it must be noted that multicollinearity may affect the standard errors of some independent variables in a regression equation without affecting the standard errors of other independent variables in the same equation. For example, if we have a multiple regression equation with four independent variables, only two of which are highly correlated with one another, only the standard errors of the partial regression coefficients for the two highly correlated variables will be affected by multicollinearity. If we delete one of the two highly correlated independent variables from the regression equation, we can expect the partial regression coefficient of the other independent variable and its standard error to change substantially. However, to the extent that the other independent variables in this multiple regression equation are uncorrelated with the two highly correlated independent variables, the partial regression coefficients of the uncorrelated independent variables and their standard errors will remain relatively unchanged.

An alternative technique for circumventing the problem of multicollinearity by respecifying the multiple regression equation involves the creation of a composite measure. In this approach, two or more highly correlated independent variables are combined into a single composite measure. Once again, this technique presumes that the highly correlated independent variables are essentially redundant measures of the same underlying theoretical construct. For example, we might have a multiple regression equation in which both income and savings are independent variables. We can expect that these two independent variables will be highly correlated with one another. Rather than including both variables in the same multiple regression equation, and introducing multicollinearity into the analysis, we might combine them into a single measure composite representing economic capital. Indeed, there are reasons to believe that this composite measure would be a more reliable measure of economic capital than either income or savings separately. The main difficulty with this approach is that it presumes that the variables in the composite measure have the same unit of measurement. In this particular example, both income and savings are measured in the same unit of measurement: dollars. However, if two or more independent variables have different units of measurement, it is necessary to convert them to standard form before using them in a composite measure.

CHAPTER 38

Assumptions of Ordinary
Least-Squares Estimation

The regression model can be used to describe the relationships between two or more variables in a sample without making any assumptions except that the dependent variable is continuous and that the relationships between these variables are linear. As a result, regression models can be used almost anytime in a purely descriptive manner to summarize the relationships between the variables in a sample. However, it is not possible to make valid statistical inferences about population parameters from sample statistics without making at least some assumptions. After all, statisticians must make certain assumptions about the characteristics of a population in order to derive the sampling distributions of the sample statistics drawn from that population. Fortunately, most of the assumptions associated with regression analysis are relatively weak in the sense that they are quite reasonable in most cases.

In terms of statistical inference, regression analysis is concerned with the parameters of the regression equation that obtains between two or more variables in the population. Moreover, the assumptions that we must make for purposes of statistical inference involve the characteristics of the population and not those of the sample. Consequently, these assumptions cannot be tested directly. However, assuming that we have a random sample drawn from this population, we can sometimes detect probable violations of these assumptions by examining the sample regression function. To simplify matters, we shall discuss the assumptions of the regression model and the ordinary least-squares estimates of its parameters in terms of simple regression with a single independent variable. However, these assumptions can readily be extended to the case of multiple regression analysis with two or more independent variables. To simplify matters even further, all of these assumptions are stated in terms of the characteristics of the errors of prediction. Collectively, these assumptions are known as the Gauss-Markov conditions.

The Gauss-Markov conditions are important because we are at risk of making invalid statistical inferences about the population regression equation whenever they are violated. Indeed, failure to satisfy these assumptions usually introduces some form of bias into our results. Some violations of these assumptions result in biased parameter estimates. Whenever our sample estimate of a population parameter is biased, the average of all possible sample estimates will not be equal to this population parameter. Other violations of these assumptions result in biased estimates of the standard errors of a sample statistic. Whenever our estimate of the standard error of a sample statistic is biased, we are unable to make any valid statistical inferences about the probability of such a sample statistic under the null hypothesis. As we shall see, the most common violations of the Gauss-Markov conditions do not usually bias the ordinary least-squares estimates of the parameters of the population regression equation, but they do introduce bias into our estimates of their standard errors. Fortunately, it is often possible to infer the direction of this bias.

The first assumption is that the expected value or mean of the errors of prediction in the population regression function is equal to zero. In short, some of the errors of prediction may be positive and others may be negative, but the mean value of these errors must be equal to zero. Mathematically, this assumption can be stated as follows:

$$\text{Mean}(u_i) = 0$$

This is a relatively minor assumption because it is not unreasonable to assume that the average error of prediction in the population regression function is zero, especially if this error represents the sum of the effects of a large number of relatively insignificant independent variables that have been inadvertently excluded from the model. In other words, it is not unreasonable to assume that all of the excluded variables in a regression model cancel one another out so that the mean of the sum of these excluded variables is equal to zero. Moreover, the consequences of violating this assumption are not especially problematic if the regression equation contains an intercept, because any systematic component to the errors of prediction will be incorporated into the sample intercept. Consequently, violations of this assumption will not introduce any bias into our sample estimate of the population regression coefficient or our estimate of the standard error of this sample regression coefficient. Only our sample estimate of the population intercept will biased.

The second assumption is that the variance of the errors of prediction is constant for all values of the independent variable. This assumption is usually referred to as the homoscedasticity condition. The term "homoscedastic" literally means "same spread." In other words, it is assumed that the errors of prediction are not related to the values of the independent variable. Mathematically, this assumption can be stated as follows:

$$\text{Var}(u_i) \;=\; \sigma_u^2 \;\text{ for all } i$$

This assumption is violated whenever the variance of the errors of prediction is not the same for all values of the independent variable. For example, the variance of a dependent variable is often directly related to the value of an independent variable. Consequently, the variance of the errors of prediction will not be the same for all values of the independent variable.

It might be noted that heteroscedasticity does not introduce any bias into of the ordinary least-squares estimate of the regression coefficient. In short, the sample regression coefficient will still provide an unbiased estimate of the population regression coefficient. However, heteroscedasticity does bias our estimate of the standard error of this sample regression coefficient. Specifically, a positive relationship between the independent variable and the variance of the errors of prediction will lead us to underestimate the actual standard error of the sample regression coefficient. As a result, we are likely to infer that a regression coefficient is significantly different than zero when, in fact, it is not. Conversely, a negative relationship between the independent variable and the variance of the errors will lead us to overestimate the actual standard error of the sample regression coefficient. Heteroscedasticity is a real problem because a positive relationship between an independent variable and the variance of the errors of prediction is not that uncommon in certain situations.

The third assumption is that the errors of prediction are independent of one another. In other words, it is assumed that the error of prediction for any observation cannot be predicted from the error of prediction for any other observation. For our purposes, this assumption can be stated mathematically as follows:

$$\text{Cov}(u_i, u_j) = 0 \text{ for all } i \text{ and } j$$

Specifically, this assumption states that the covariance of the errors of prediction is equal to zero. This assumption is sometimes violated in the case of time-series data because the error of prediction at a given point in time, t, is often related to the error of prediction at the previous point in time, $t - 1$. This occurs because the excluded variables that produce an error in one direction at one point in time are likely to be present, at least to some extent, at the next point in time. Under these conditions, the errors of prediction become serially correlated over time. This situation is known as autocorrelation.

It is important to understand how the presence of autocorrelated error affects the ordinary least-squares estimates of the regression model. To begin with, the sample regression coefficient still provides an unbiased estimate of the population regression coefficient in the presence of autocorrelation. However, autocorrelation does produce a biased estimate of the standard error of the sample regression coefficient, which might lead us to make an incorrect statistical inference. If the autocorrelation is positive, the estimate of the standard error of the sample regression coefficient will underestimate the actual standard error. As a result, we are likely to conclude that a regression coefficient is statistically significant when, in fact, it is not. Conversely, negative autocorrelation will lead us to overestimate the actual standard error of the sample regression coefficient. Autocorrelation is a real problem because a positive serial correlation between the errors of prediction is not that uncommon in models employing time-series data.

The fourth assumption is that the errors of prediction and the independent variable are independent. In other words, it is assumed that the error of prediction for an observation cannot be predicted by its value on the independent variable. For our purposes, this assumption can be stated mathematically as follows:

$$\text{Cov}(u_i, x_i) = 0$$

This assumption can be violated in a number of ways. To begin with, it is violated whenever an independent variable contains a significant amount of measurement error. Although measurement error in the dependent variable is not especially problematic, measurement error in the independent variable will introduce a degree of bias into the regression coefficient. Next, this assumption is violated whenever we have excluded an independent variable that is highly correlated both with the dependent variable and with the other independent variables. This is essentially the problem of specification error. Finally, this assumption is violated whenever there is reciprocal causation such that the dependent variable has an effect on the independent variable. This situation is referred to as "simultaneity." In general, sample estimates of the population regression coefficient will be biased whenever this assumption has been violated. Simultaneity also affects the accuracy of the estimates of the sampling error of the sample regression coefficient.

Finally, even if our estimates of the intercept and the regression coefficient, as well as their standard errors, are unbiased, we must make additional assumptions in order to specify the exact sampling distribution of these sample statistics. In particular, we need to know the sampling distribution of the intercept and the regression coefficient if we wish to employ statistical tests such as the t test or the F test. It will be recalled that the central limit theorem assures us that the sampling distribution of the mean of a variable is normal, even if the variable itself does not have a normal distribution. Fortunately, the central limit theorem can be readily generalized to both the intercept and the regression coefficient. Specifically, both the intercept and the regression coefficient are normally distributed in the case of large samples, even if the dependent and independent variables are not normally distributed. However, the central limit theorem only applies to large samples. In the case of relatively small samples, the intercept and the regression coefficient will not be normally distributed unless the errors of prediction are normally distributed. This is not an unreasonable assumption if we believe that the errors of prediction capture the overall effects of a large number of excluded independent variables. Indeed, there is considerable evidence that statistical tests such as the t test and F test yield valid inferences, even in relatively small samples, whenever the errors of prediction have a symmetric distribution that approximates a normal distribution.

CHAPTER 39

Beyond Ordinary
Regression Analysis

In response to the various problems that arise whenever the assumptions required by ordinary least-squares estimation procedures cannot be met, statisticians have developed a series of special estimation procedures. It will be recalled that most of the problems associated with violations of these assumptions involve biases in the standard errors of the parameters of the regression model. In other words, we can rely on ordinary least-squares estimation procedures to provide us with valuable information about the direction and magnitude of the parameters of the regression model, even if we cannot rely on the estimated standard errors of these parameter estimates for purposes of statistical inference. However, if we wish to make valid statistical inferences, based on unbiased estimates of the standard errors of these parameter estimates, we must be prepared to employ special estimation procedures that are appropriate to the problem at hand. Most of these special estimation procedures yield what are known as "consistent" estimates of the parameters of the regression model. Strictly speaking, consistent estimates are not unbiased, but their bias is relatively small in large samples. Moreover, these consistent estimates have relatively large standard errors, even if these estimates of the standard errors are unbiased. The details of these special estimation procedures can be found in advanced statistical and econometric textbooks. However, it is possible to provide an overview of the essential logic underlying each of these estimation procedures.

One of the often overlooked but most common violations of the assumptions required for ordinary least-squares estimation involves *heteroscedasticity*. As noted earlier, this a serious problem because, whenever the variance of the errors of prediction is positively related to the independent variable, ordinary least-squares procedures will underestimate the actual standard error of a regression coefficient. We can assess the degree of heteroscedasticity in a regression model by examining a scatter plot of the errors of prediction for each predicted value of the dependent variable. Another technique for identifying heteroscedasticity is to compare the error variances of the observations with the largest predicted values on the dependent variable with the error variances of the observations with the smallest predicted values. Sometimes we can reduce the degree of heteroscedasticity in a model by transforming one or more of the variables using a nonlinear transformation in order to reduce the magnitude of extreme values on those variables. However, if we cannot avoid heteroscedasticity in this manner, we can correct for its effects by using a special estimation procedure known as *weighted least-squares*. In this procedure, each observation is "weighted" in the course of estimating the parameters of the regression equation. Moreover, the "weight" of each observation in the regression analysis is inversely proportional to its error variance. In short, those observations with the smallest error variance receive the greatest weight in calculating the parameters of the regression equation, whereas those observations with the largest error variance receive the least weight. In practice, this procedure typically involves the use of a "scale variable" that is highly correlated with the variance of the errors of prediction. Once we have identified such a scale variable, we can divide the values of the observations on all of the variables by the value of the associated observation on this scale variable.

Another important violation of the assumptions required for ordinary least-squares estimation involves *autocorrelation*. In general, we must consider the possibility of autocorrelation whenever we have time-series data. This is a serious problem because, whenever the errors of prediction are positively correlated with one another over time, ordinary least-squares procedures underestimate the actual standard error of a regression coefficient. We can determine the degree of autocorrelation by computing the serial correlation among the errors of prediction. In short, we compute the correlation between the error of prediction in each time period with the error of prediction in the previous time period. Indeed, there is a special statistical test, known as the Durbin-Watson test, which enables us to determine whether or not autocorrelation is a serious problem. If we conclude that significant autocorrelation is present in our analysis, we can correct for its effects using a special estimation procedure known as *generalized least-squares*. In this procedure, each observation is "adjusted" in the course of estimating the parameters of the regression equation. Specifically, each observation is replaced by a residual observation that has had the effects of autocorrelation removed from it. In short, each observation is "residualized" with respect to the observation on that variable for the previous year and the degree of autocorrelation over time.

A third important violation of the assumptions required for ordinary least-squares estimation involves *simultaneity*. This is a very serious problem because, whenever the dependent variable has an effect on one of the independent variables in a regression model, ordinary least-squares procedures will provide us with parameter estimates that are biased as well as biased estimates of the standard errors of these parameter estimates. However, we can obtain unbiased estimates of the parameters of the regression model and unbiased estimates of their standard errors if we employ a special estimation procedure known as *two-stage least-squares*. As the names implies, this is a two-stage estimation procedure. In the first stage, we regress the independent variable that is affected by the dependent variable on one or more exogenous variables that are not affected by the dependent variable. In the second stage, we replace the independent variable in question with an "instrumental variable" which represents only that component of this independent variable that is predicted by the exogenous independent variables. In short, this procedure attempts to "purify" the independent variable of the effects of the dependent variable by removing from it any variance that cannot be explained by the exogenous variables. Since the exogenous variables are unaffected by the dependent variable, the instrumental variable constructed using these exogenous variables is also unaffected by the dependent variable. In order to employ this procedure, we must be able to identify one or more exogenous variables that are not independent variables in the regression equation in question but are good predictors of the independent variable subject to simultaneity.

In addition to these assumptions, there is one other assumption required of regression models estimated using ordinary least-squares estimation procedures. This assumption is so fundamental that it has been largely implicit to this point. Specifically, regression analysis using ordinary least-squares estimation procedures assumes that the dependent variable is continuous. However, there are many situations in which we are interested in dependent variables that are categorical. In many cases, these categorical variables are simple dichotomies that can be represented by binary variables. For example, we might be interested in examining the effect of income on whether an individual voted for a particular political candidate. At first glance, it might seem that such an analysis could be accomplished using an ordinary regression model with a binary dependent variable. For example, we might consider estimating the parameters of a regression equation in which the dependent variable was coded as either a one or a zero. Although it is possible to compute the parameters of such a regression model using ordinary least-squares estimation procedures, these parameter estimates lack many of the statistical properties typically associated with ordinary least-squares regression analysis. This type of regression model is know as a *linear probability model.*

Unfortunately, linear probability models are not very useful for the purposes of statistical inference. Although ordinary least-squares estimation procedures will yield parameter estimates that are unbiased, the standard errors of these parameter estimates will be biased. This situation arises because regression models with binary dependent variables invariably contain substantial heteroscedasticity. Whenever we use a continuous variable to predict a binary variable, we are likely to obtain large errors of prediction whenever the continuous independent variable is large in absolute terms. Consequently, we will not be able to determine the statistical significance of the intercept or the regression coefficient. Moreover, the use of ordinary least-squares estimation procedures in regression models with binary dependent variables can yield predicted scores on the binary dependent variable that are smaller than zero and larger than one. Once again, this is likely to happen whenever the continuous independent variable is large in absolute terms. The most appropriate solution to this problem is to employ *logistic regression analysis.*

Logistic regression analysis was developed precisely for the purpose of estimating the parameters of regression models with binary dependent variables. Although logistic regression analysis has the same mathematical form as ordinary regression analysis, it is a very different statistical technique. For example, in logistic regression analysis the dependent variable is actually the value of the natural logarithm of the odds that the dependent binary variable is equal to one rather than zero. Moreover, in order to estimate the parameters of this logistic regression model, it is necessary to employ maximum-likelihood estimation procedures. Maximum-likelihood estimation is based on a different logic than ordinary least-squares estimation. Moreover, once the parameters of the logistic regression model have been estimated using maximum-likelihood procedures, it is not an easy matter to interpret these parameters. Indeed, the parameters of a logistic regression equation are typically interpreted as the expected change in the "log of the odds" of the dependent variable. Even if we simplify the interpretation of the parameters of the logistic regression model by taking the antilogarithms of these values, it is still only possible to interpret these transformed parameters in terms of the expected change in the "odds" of the binary dependent variable associated with a one unit change in the independent variable. Logistic regression analysis is a powerful statistical procedure for conducting regression analysis with binary dependent variables. However, logistic regression analysis is more difficult to learn and to interpret than ordinary regression analysis. The only simple alternative is to avoid the problem of categorical dependent variables by developing continuous measures of those variables whenever possible.

APPENDIX A

Derivation of the Mean and Variance of a Linear Function

Regression analysis is based on the use of linear functions. Indeed, the predicted value of the dependent variable in a regression model is a linear function of the values of the independent variables. As a result, it is possible to compute the mean and variance of the predicted value of the dependent variable directly from the means and variances of the independent variables in a regression equation. In vector notation, the equation for the predicted value of the dependent variable, in the case of a multiple regression equation with two independent variables, is given by:

$$\hat{y} \;=\; \mathbf{u}a \;+\; \mathbf{x}_1 b_1 \;+\; \mathbf{x}_2 b_2$$

Using this equation, it is a relatively simple matter to derive the mean of the predicted values of the dependent variable from the means of the independent variables, the regression coefficients for these variables, and the intercept.

To begin with, it will be recalled that the mean of a variable, using vector algebra, is given by:

$$\text{Mean}(\hat{y}) \;=\; \frac{1}{N}\,(\mathbf{u}'\hat{y})$$

The product of these two vectors in this equation can be simplified as follows:

$$\mathbf{u'\hat{y}} = \mathbf{u'(ua + x_1 b_1 + x_2 b_2)}$$

$$= \mathbf{u'ua + u'x_1 b_1 + u'x_2 b_2}$$

$$= \mathrm{Na} + \sum x_{1i}\, b_1 + \sum x_{2i}\, b_2$$

$$= \mathrm{Na} + b_1 \sum x_{1i} + b_2 \sum x_{2i}$$

$$= \mathrm{Na} + b_1 \mathrm{N}\,\bar{x}_1 + b_2 \mathrm{N}\,\bar{x}_2$$

This quantity can be substituted into the equation for the mean of a variable such that:

$$\mathrm{Mean}(\hat{y}) = \frac{1}{\mathrm{N}}\,(\mathbf{u'\hat{y}}) = \frac{1}{\mathrm{N}}\,(\mathrm{Na} + b_1 \mathrm{N}\,\bar{x}_1 + b_2 \mathrm{N}\,\bar{x}_2)$$

$$= a + b_1\,\bar{x}_1 + b_2\,\bar{x}_2$$

Therefore, the mean of the predicted value of the dependent variable is a function of the means of the independent variables, their regression coefficients, and the intercept.

The variance of the predicted value of the dependent variable can be derived in a similar manner. However, we can greatly simplify this derivation by introducing the assumption that both the dependent variable and the independent variables have means that are equal to zero. This simplifying assumption is of no real consequence because the variance of a variable, which is the average squared deviation from the mean, is unaffected by the value of the mean itself. Moreover, because of the manner in which the intercept is computed, the mean of the predicted value of the dependent variable will be equal to zero whenever the mean of the dependent variable is equal to zero. Consequently, the sum of squares of the predicted values of the dependent variable is given by:

$$\mathrm{SS}(\hat{y}) = (\hat{y} - \bar{y})'(\hat{y} - \bar{y}) = \hat{y}'\hat{y}$$

$$= (\mathbf{x_1 b_1 + x_2 b_2})'(\mathbf{x_1 b_1 + x_2 b_2})$$

$$= b_1 \mathbf{x_1'}(\mathbf{x_1 b_1 + x_2 b_2}) + b_2 \mathbf{x_2'}(\mathbf{x_1 b_1 + x_2 b_2})$$

$$= b_1 x_1' x_1 b_1 + b_1 x_1' x_2 b_2 + b_2 x_2' x_1 b_1 + b_2 x_2' x_2 b_2$$

This equation can be simplified even further by noting the following equivalencies:

$$b_1 x_1' x_1 b_1 = b_1^2 x_1' x_1 = b_1^2 \sum x_{1i}^2$$

$$b_2 x_2' x_2 b_2 = b_2^2 x_2' x_2 = b_2^2 \sum x_{2i}^2$$

$$b_1 x_1' x_2 b_2 = b_2 x_2' x_1 b_1 = b_1 b_2 x_1 x_2 = b_1 b_2 \sum x_{1i} x_{2i}$$

As a result, the sum of squares of the predicted values of the dependent variable is given by:

$$SS(\hat{y}) = b_1^2 \sum x_{1i}^2 + b_2^2 \sum x_{2i}^2 + 2 b_1 b_2 \sum x_{1i} x_{2i}$$

Therefore, we can derive the variance of the predicted value of the dependent variable as follows:

$$Var(\hat{y}) = \frac{1}{N}(b_1^2 \sum x_{1i}^2) + \frac{1}{N}(b_2^2 \sum x_{2i}^2) +$$

$$\frac{1}{N} 2(b_1 b_2 \sum x_{1i} x_{2i})$$

$$= b_1^2 \frac{1}{N} \sum x_{1i}^2 + b_2^2 \frac{1}{N} \sum x_{2i}^2 +$$

$$2 b_1 b_2 \frac{1}{N} \sum x_{1i} x_{2i}$$

Of course, this equation can be reduced to a series of more familiar quantities as follows:

$$Var(\hat{y}) = b_1^2 Var(x_1) + b_2^2 Var(x_2) + 2 b_1 b_2 Cov(x_1, x_2)$$

In other words, the variance of the predicted value of the dependent variable is a function of the regression coefficients of the independent variables, the variances of the independent variables, and the covariance between these independent variables. This equation can readily be expanded to obtain the variance of the predicted value of the dependent variable whenever there are more than two independent variables. For example, in the case of three independent variables, there are three terms involving the variances and regression coefficients of each of these independent variables and three terms involving the regression coefficients of these independent variables and the covariances between each pair of independent variables.

Finally, it must be noted that this equation has a special interpretation whenever all of the variables are expressed in standard form such that both the dependent and independent variables have variances that are equal to one. Specifically, in this case, the variance of the predicted values of the dependent variable is given by:

$$\text{Var}(\hat{z}_y) = b_1^{*2} \text{Var}(z_1) + b_2^{*2} \text{Var}(z_2) + 2 b_1^* b_2^* \text{Cov}(z_1, z_2)$$

$$= b_1^{*2} + b_2^{*2} + 2 b_1^* b_2^* r_{12}$$

Moreover, it will be recalled that the coefficient of determination is equal to the ratio of the variance of the predicted value of the dependent variable to the variance of the observed value of that variable such that:

$$R_{y.12}^2 = \frac{\text{Var}(\hat{y})}{\text{Var}(y)} = \frac{\text{Var}(\hat{z}_y)}{\text{Var}(z_y)} = \text{Var}(\hat{z}_y)$$

$$= b_1^{*2} + b_2^{*2} + 2 b_1^* b_2^* r_{12}$$

In short, the coefficient of determination can be computed directly from the standardized regression coefficients of the independent variables and the correlations among these independent variables.

APPENDIX B

Derivation of the Least-Squares Regression Coefficient

The derivation of the least-squares regression coefficient requires some familiarity with calculus. From a mathematical point of view, the main problem posed by regression analysis involves the estimation of a regression coefficient and an intercept that minimize some function of the errors of prediction. The least-squares estimation procedure adopts a solution to this problem that is based on minimizing the sum of the squared errors of prediction. This criterion can be stated algebraically as follows:

$$\text{Minimize SS(e)} = \sum e_i^2 = \sum (y_i - \hat{y}_i)^2$$

where

$$\hat{y}_i = a + bx_i$$

Obviously, the values of the predicted scores and, therefore, the values of the errors of prediction are determined by the choice of a particular intercept and regression coefficient.

If we substitute this linear function for the predicted value of the dependent variable, the problem becomes one of finding the regression coefficient, b, and the intercept, a, that minimize the following function:

$$S(a,b) = \sum (y_i - a - bx_i)^2$$

In order to minimize this function, we calculate the partial derivatives of both b and a using the chain rule of differentiation and the rule that the derivative of a sum is equal to the sum of the derivatives as follows:

$$\frac{\partial S}{\partial b} = \sum 2(y_i - a - bx_i)(-x_i)$$

$$\frac{\partial S}{\partial a} = \sum 2(y_i - a - bx_i)(-1)$$

Performing the indicated multiplication, dividing both partial derivatives by -2, and setting them both equal to zero, we obtain:

$$\sum(-x_i y_i + bx_i^2 + ax_i) = 0$$

$$\sum(-y_i + bx_i + a) = 0$$

Rearranging the terms in these equations, we obtain:

$$b\sum x_i^2 - \sum x_i y_i + a\sum x_i = 0$$

$$aN - \sum y_i + b\sum x_i = 0$$

These equations can be greatly simplified if we assume, for the sake of simplicity and without loss of generality, that the independent variable, x, is expressed in mean deviation form such that:

$$\sum x_i = 0$$

Specifically, under this assumption, these equations reduce to:

$$b = \frac{\sum x_i y_i}{\sum x_i^2}$$

$$a = \frac{\sum y_i}{N} = \bar{y}$$

If we divide both the numerator and the denominator of the equation for b by N, we obtain the more familiar equation for the least-squares regression coefficient as the covariance of two variables divided by the variance of the independent variable:

$$b = \frac{\text{Cov}(x,y)}{\text{Var}(x)}$$

Moreover, the equation for a, whenever the independent variable is expressed in mean deviation form, is simply a special case of the more general equation for the intercept such that:

$$a = \bar{y} - b\bar{x}$$

where

$$\bar{x} = 0$$

This result obtains because the mean of any variable expressed in mean deviation form is zero. The least-squares intercept insures that the predicted value of the dependent variable is equal to the mean of the dependent variable whenever the independent variable is equal to its mean. This result is obvious if we simply rearrange the equation for the intercept as follows:

$$\bar{y} = a + b\bar{x}$$

These results were obtained using the simplifying assumption that the independent variable is expressed in mean deviation form. However, it can be demonstrated that this assumption is not necessary to obtain these equations. Indeed, the covariance between two variables and the variance of the independent variable are the same whether or not the independent variable is expressed in mean deviation form.

APPENDIX C

Derivation of the Standard Error of
the Simple Regression Coefficient

In order to test for the significance of a regression coefficient, we must be able to estimate its standard error. We begin with the generic equation for the simple regression coefficient as a ratio of the covariance between two variables to the variance of the independent variable such that:

$$b = \frac{Cov(x,y)}{Var(x)}$$

For the sake of simplicity and without loss of generality, we shall assume that both the dependent variable, y, and the independent variable, x, are expressed in mean deviation form.

First, we multiply both the numerator and the denominator of this equation by N, the number of cases, and simplify as follows:

$$b = \frac{N\,c_{xy}}{N\,s_x^2} = \frac{\sum x_i\,y_i}{\sum x_i^2}$$

This equation can be expressed somewhat differently such that:

$$b = \frac{\sum x_i\,y_i}{\sum x_i^2} = \sum \left(\frac{x_i}{\sum x_i^2} \right) y_i$$

Consequently, the regression coefficient can be expressed as a sum of the weighted values of the dependent variable, y, as follows:

$$b = \sum w_i \, y_i$$

where

$$w_i = \frac{x_i}{\sum x_i^2}$$

In other words, the simple regression coefficient is equal to a linear function of the values of the dependent variable in which each value of the dependent variable, y, is multiplied by the ratio of the value of the corresponding independent variable, x, to its sum of squares.

Next, we wish to obtain the variance of this linear function. It can be shown that the variance of this linear function is equal to the sum of the products of the squared weights, w, and the variances of the variables in the linear function as follows:

$$\text{Var}(b) = w_i^2 \, s_{y1}^2 + w_i^2 \, s_{y2}^2 + \ldots + w_i^2 \, s_{yn}^2$$

This equation is based on two important assumptions. To begin with, we have assumed that we have repeated samples in which the values of the independent variables, x, remain fixed. This is known as the "fixed effects" assumption. This assumption would be satisfied, for example, whenever we have the same number of observations with each value of the independent variable in each sample. Moreover, we have also assumed that the values of the dependent variable, y, within each sample are independent of one another. In other words, the value of each observation on the dependent variable is not affected by the values of the other observations on the dependent variable in that sample.

In order to simplify this equation even further, we make one more important assumption. Specifically, we assume that the variance of the dependent variable, y, is the same for all values of the independent variable such that:

$$s_{y1}^2 = s_{y2}^2 = \ldots = s_{yn}^2 = s_y^2$$

This is known as the "homoscedasticity" assumption. Given this assumption, the variance of the regression coefficient can be seen to be equal to the product of the variance of the dependent variable and the sum of squared weights as follows:

$$\text{Var(b)} \;=\; \sum w_i^2 \, s_{iy}^2 \;=\; s_y^2 \sum w_i^2$$

This equation can be expressed differently as follows:

$$\text{Var(b)} \;=\; s_y^2 \sum \left(\frac{x_i}{\sum x_i^2} \right)^2 \;=\; s_y^2 \, \frac{\sum x_i^2}{\left(\sum x_i^2 \right)^2}$$

such that:

$$\text{Var(b)} \;=\; \frac{s_y^2}{\left(\sum x_i^2 \right)^2} \sum x_i^2 \;=\; \frac{s_y^2}{\sum x_i^2}$$

Consequently, it can be seen that the variance of the regression coefficient is equal to the variance of the dependent variable divided by the sum of squares of the independent variable. This equation can be expressed in more familiar terms as follows:

$$\text{Var(b)} \;=\; \frac{s_y^2}{N \, s_x^2}$$

The standard error of a statistic is equal to the square root of its variance. Therefore, the standard error of the regression coefficient is given by:

$$\text{S.D.(b)} \;=\; \sqrt{ \frac{s_y^2}{N \, s_x^2} }$$

It must be noted that, in order to obtain an unbiased estimate of the standard error of the regression coefficient, we must adjust for the number of degrees of freedom as follows:

$$s_b = \sqrt{\dfrac{s_y^2}{(N-2)\, s_x^2}}$$

This is, of course, the familiar equation for the standard error of the regression coefficient.

It might be noted that the equation for the regression coefficient as a linear function of the values of the dependent variable tells us a great deal about how the value of the regression coefficient is affected by the values of the dependent variable and the independent variable. Once again, the simple regression coefficient is given by:

$$b = \left(\frac{x_1}{\sum x_i^2}\right) y_1 + \left(\frac{x_2}{\sum x_i^2}\right) y_2 + \dots + \left(\frac{x_n}{\sum x_i^2}\right) y_n$$

Consequently, the contribution of any observation to the value of the regression coefficient is determined both by its deviation from the mean on the independent variable and by its deviation from the mean on the dependent variable.

Finally, this derivation of the standard error of the simple regression coefficient was based on a series of assumptions that comprise the "fixed effects regression model." It turns out that some of these assumptions are overly restrictive, especially the assumption that we have the same number of observations with each value of the independent variable in repeated samples. This assumption can be relaxed if we are willing to assume that the values of the independent variables are independent of their respective errors of prediction. However, we must continue to assume that the variance of the dependent variable, or at least the variance of the errors of prediction, is constant over the different values of the independent variable. This "homoscedasticity" assumption is essential if ordinary least-squares estimations procedures are to yield unbiased estimates of the standard errors of the parameter estimates.

Derivation of the Normal Equations

As with the derivation of the least-squares regression coefficient, the derivation of the normal equations for the least-squares standardized partial regression coefficients requires some familiarity with calculus. We begin with the matrix algebra equation for the multiple regression model, where we have assumed, for the sake of simplicity and without loss of generality, that all of the variables are in mean deviation form, such that:

$$y = Xb + e$$

This assumption, that all of the variables are expressed as deviations from their means, eliminates the intercept from the multiple regression equation.

Next, we can obtain the matrix algebra equation for the sum of squared error as follows:

$$e = y - Xb$$

The problem becomes one of finding the vector of partial regression coefficients, b, that minimizes the following function:

$$S(b) = e'e = (y - Xb)'(y - Xb)$$

This equation can be expanded as follows:

$$S(b) = y'y - y'Xb - (Xb)'y + (Xb)'Xb$$

It must be noted that $y'Xb$ is a scalar product and that it is identical to $(Xb)'y$. Consequently, these two scalar products can be collected together to yield:

$$S(b) = y'y - 2y'Xb + b'X'Xb$$

This function can be minimized by differentiating this equation with respect to b and equating the derivatives to zero. First, it can be shown that the vector of partial derivatives is given by:

$$\frac{\partial S}{\partial b} = 0 - 2X'y + 2X'Xb$$

Of course, this result is based on the derivatives of linear and quadratic forms. Next, we can simplify these partial derivatives and set them equal to zero as follows:

$$X'y - X'Xb = 0$$

This equation can be solved to obtain the vector of partial regression coefficients such that:

$$b = (X'X)^{-1}X'y$$

It must be noted that the first quantity on the right, $X'X^{-1}$, is simply the inverse of the matrix whose main diagonal elements are the sums of squares of the independent variables and whose off-diagonal elements are the sums of the cross-products of the independent variables. Similarly, the second quantity on the right, $X'y$, is the column vector of the sum of the cross-products of the independent variables and the dependent variable. Therefore, the vector of partial regression coefficients, b, is equivalent to the inverse of the variance-covariance matrix of the independent variables, C_{xx}^{-1}, postmultiplied by the vector of covariances between the independent variables and the dependent variable, c_{yx}, such that:

$$b = C_{xx}^{-1}c_{yx}$$

Moreover, whenever all of the variables are in standard form so that their variances are equal to one, the covariances among the variables become correlations such that this equation reduces to:

$$\mathbf{b}^* = \mathbf{R}_{xx}^{-1}\, \mathbf{r}_{yx}$$

This result gives us the equation for the standardized partial regression coefficient.

Although the matrix algebra equation for the partial regression coefficients, derived from the normal equations, is rather complicated, it is analogous to the equation for the simple regression coefficient. Indeed, if multiplication by the inverse of a matrix is the matrix algebra analog to division in ordinary algebra, the equation for the partial regression coefficients can be viewed as the ratio of a function of the covariances between the dependent variable and the independent variables to a function of the variances and covariances of the independent variables.

APPENDIX E

Statistical Tables

Table 1. Critical Values of t (Two-tailed Test)

d.f.	Probability Level				
	0.20	0.10	0.05	0.01	0.001
5	1.476	2.015	2.571	4.032	6.859
6	1.440	1.943	2.447	3.707	5.959
7	1.415	1.895	2.365	3.499	5.405
8	1.397	1.860	2.306	3.355	5.041
9	1.383	1.833	2.262	3.250	4.781
10	1.372	1.812	2.228	3.169	4.587
11	1.363	1.796	2.201	3.106	4.437
12	1.356	1.782	2.179	3.055	4.318
13	1.350	1.771	2.160	3.012	4.221
14	1.345	1.761	2.145	2.977	4.140
15	1.341	1.753	2.131	2.947	4.073
16	1.337	1.746	2.120	2.921	4.015
17	1.333	1.740	2.110	2.898	3.965
18	1.330	1.734	2.101	2.878	3.922
19	1.328	1.729	2.093	2.861	3.883
20	1.325	1.725	2.086	2.845	3.850
21	1.323	1.721	2.080	2.831	3.819
22	1.321	1.717	2.074	2.819	3.792
23	1.319	1.714	2.069	2.807	3.767
24	1.318	1.711	2.064	2.797	3.745
25	1.316	1.708	2.060	2.787	3.725
26	1.315	1.706	2.056	2.779	3.707
27	1.314	1.703	2.052	2.771	3.690
28	1.313	1.701	2.048	2.763	3.674
29	1.311	1.699	2.045	2.756	3.659
30	1.310	1.697	2.042	2.750	3.646
40	1.303	1.684	2.021	2.704	3.551
60	1.296	1.671	2.000	2.660	3.460
120	1.289	1.658	1.980	2.617	3.373
∞	1.282	1.645	1.960	2.576	3.291

Table 2. Critical Values of F (0.05 Probability Level)

denom-inator d.f.	numerator d.f.							
	1	2	3	4	5	6	7	8
5	6.61	5.79	5.41	5.19	5.05	4.95	4.88	4.82
6	5.99	5.14	4.76	4.53	4.39	4.28	4.21	4.15
7	5.59	4.74	4.35	4.12	3.97	3.87	3.79	3.73
8	5.32	4.46	4.07	3.84	3.69	3.58	3.50	3.44
9	5.12	4.26	3.86	3.63	3.48	3.37	3.29	3.23
10	4.96	4.10	3.71	3.48	3.33	3.22	3.14	3.07
11	4.84	3.98	3.59	3.36	3.20	3.09	3.01	2.95
12	4.75	3.88	3.49	3.26	3.11	3.00	2.91	2.85
13	4.67	3.80	3.41	3.18	3.02	2.92	2.83	2.77
14	4.60	3.74	3.34	3.11	2.96	2.85	2.76	2.70
15	4.54	3.68	3.29	3.06	2.90	2.79	2.71	2.64
16	4.49	3.63	3.24	3.01	2.85	2.74	2.66	2.59
17	4.45	3.59	3.20	2.96	2.81	2.70	2.61	2.55
18	4.41	3.55	3.16	2.93	2.77	2.66	2.58	2.51
19	4.38	3.52	3.13	2.90	2.74	2.63	2.54	2.48
20	4.35	3.49	3.10	2.87	2.71	2.60	2.51	2.45
21	4.32	3.47	3.07	2.84	2.68	2.57	2.49	2.42
22	4.30	3.44	3.05	2.82	2.66	2.55	2.46	2.40
23	4.28	3.42	3.03	2.80	2.64	2.53	2.44	2.38
24	4.26	3.40	3.01	2.78	2.62	2.51	2.42	2.36
25	4.24	3.38	2.99	2.76	2.60	2.49	2.40	2.34
26	4.22	3.37	2.98	2.74	2.59	2.47	2.39	2.32
27	4.21	3.35	2.96	2.73	2.57	2.46	2.37	2.30
28	4.20	3.34	2.95	2.71	2.56	2.44	2.36	2.29
29	4.18	3.33	2.93	2.70	2.54	2.43	2.35	2.28
30	4.17	3.32	2.92	2.69	2.53	2.42	2.33	2.27
40	4.08	3.23	2.84	2.61	2.45	2.34	2.25	2.18
60	4.00	3.15	2.76	2.52	2.37	2.25	2.17	2.10
120	3.92	3.07	2.68	2.45	2.29	2.17	2.09	2.02
∞	3.84	2.99	2.60	2.37	2.21	2.09	2.01	1.94

Table 3. Critical Values of F (0.01 Probability Level)

denom-inator d.f.	numerator d.f.							
	1	2	3	4	5	6	7	8
5	16.26	13.27	12.06	11.39	10.97	10.67	10.46	10.27
6	13.74	10.92	9.78	9.15	8.75	8.47	8.26	8.10
7	12.25	9.55	8.45	7.85	7.46	7.19	6.99	6.84
8	11.26	8.65	7.59	7.01	6.63	6.37	6.18	6.03
9	10.56	8.02	6.99	6.42	6.06	5.80	5.61	5.47
10	10.04	7.56	6.55	5.99	5.64	5.39	5.20	5.06
11	9.65	7.20	6.22	5.67	5.32	5.07	4.89	4.74
12	9.33	6.93	5.95	5.41	5.06	4.82	4.64	4.50
13	9.07	6.70	5.74	5.20	4.86	4.62	4.44	4.30
14	8.86	6.51	5.56	5.03	4.69	4.46	4.28	4.14
15	8.68	6.36	5.42	4.89	4.56	4.32	4.14	4.00
16	8.53	6.23	5.29	4.77	4.44	4.20	4.03	3.89
17	8.40	6.11	5.18	4.67	4.34	4.10	3.93	3.79
18	8.28	6.01	5.09	4.58	4.25	4.01	3.84	3.71
19	8.18	5.93	5.01	4.50	4.17	3.94	3.77	3.63
20	8.10	5.85	4.94	4.43	4.10	3.87	3.70	3.56
21	8.02	5.78	4.87	4.37	4.04	3.81	3.64	3.51
22	7.94	5.72	4.82	4.31	3.99	3.76	3.59	3.45
23	7.88	5.66	4.76	4.26	3.94	3.71	3.54	3.41
24	7.82	5.61	4.72	4.22	3.90	3.67	3.50	3.36
25	7.77	5.57	4.68	4.18	3.86	3.63	3.46	3.32
26	7.72	5.53	4.64	4.14	3.82	3.59	3.42	3.29
27	7.68	5.49	4.60	4.11	3.78	3.56	3.39	3.26
28	7.64	5.45	4.57	4.07	3.75	3.53	3.36	3.23
29	7.60	5.42	4.54	4.04	3.73	3.50	3.33	3.20
30	7.56	5.39	4.51	4.02	3.70	3.47	3.30	3.17
40	7.31	5.18	4.31	3.83	3.51	3.29	3.12	2.99
60	7.08	4.98	4.13	3.65	3.34	3.12	2.95	2.82
120	6.85	4.79	3.95	3.48	3.17	2.96	2.79	2.66
∞	6.63	4.60	3.78	3.32	3.02	2.80	2.64	2.51

Table 4. Critical Values of F (0.001 Probability Level)

denom-inator d.f.	numerator d.f.							
	1	2	3	4	5	6	7	8
5	47.04	36.61	33.20	31.09	29.75	28.83	28.16	27.65
6	35.51	27.00	23.70	21.90	20.81	20.03	19.46	19.03
7	29.22	21.69	18.77	17.19	16.21	15.52	15.02	14.63
8	25.42	18.49	15.83	14.39	13.49	12.86	12.40	12.07
9	22.86	16.39	13.90	12.56	11.71	11.13	10.70	10.37
10	21.04	14.91	12.55	11.28	10.48	9.92	9.52	9.20
11	19.69	13.81	11.56	10.35	9.58	9.05	8.66	8.35
12	18.64	12.97	10.80	9.63	8.89	8.38	8.00	7.71
13	17.81	12.31	10.21	9.07	8.35	7.86	7.49	7.21
14	17.14	11.78	9.73	8.62	7.92	7.43	7.08	6.80
15	16.59	11.34	9.34	8.25	7.57	7.09	6.74	6.47
16	16.12	10.97	9.00	7.94	7.27	6.81	6.46	6.19
17	15.72	10.66	8.73	7.68	7.02	6.56	6.22	5.96
18	15.38	10.39	8.49	7.46	6.81	6.35	6.02	5.76
19	15.08	10.16	8.28	7.26	6.61	6.18	5.85	5.59
20	14.82	9.95	8.10	7.10	6.46	6.02	5.69	5.44
21	14.59	9.77	7.94	6.95	6.32	5.88	5.56	5.31
22	14.38	9.61	7.80	6.81	6.19	5.76	5.44	5.19
23	14.19	9.47	7.67	6.69	6.08	5.65	5.33	5.09
24	14.03	9.34	7.55	6.59	5.98	5.55	5.23	4.99
25	13.88	9.22	7.45	6.49	5.88	5.46	5.15	4.91
26	13.74	9.12	7.36	6.41	5.80	5.38	5.07	4.83
27	13.61	9.02	7.27	6.33	5.73	5.31	5.00	4.76
28	13.50	8.93	7.19	6.25	5.66	5.24	4.93	4.69
29	13.39	8.85	7.12	6.19	5.59	5.18	4.87	4.64
30	13.29	8.77	7.05	6.12	5.53	5.12	4.82	4.58
40	12.61	8.25	6.60	5.70	5.13	4.73	4.44	4.21
60	11.97	7.76	6.17	5.31	4.76	4.37	4.09	3.87
120	11.38	7.31	5.79	4.95	4.42	4.04	3.77	3.55
∞	10.83	6.91	5.42	4.62	4.10	3.74	3.48	3.27

Suggested Readings

In order to simplify the presentation of the material, this textbook does not include any citations. However, the reader may find more comprehensive discussions of the essential results mentioned in this textbook in any number of more advanced statistics textbooks. Indeed, the adventurous reader may wish to pursue in more detail some of the statistical issues and methods mentioned in passing in this textbook. The following textbooks, drawn from the fields of sociology, economics and psychology, are recommended both for their accessibility to the average student of introductory statistics and for their coverage of particular topics.

BASIC STATISTICAL THEORY

Statistics by William L. Hays (Fort Worth, TX: Holt, Rinehart & Winston, 1988, 750 pages). This massive textbook is designed to provide psychologists with a comprehensive introduction to statistical methods, including simple and multiple regression. It contains an excellent discussion of the analysis of variance model and a very accessible explanation of various sampling distributions.

MULTIPLE REGRESSION AND REGRESSION DIAGNOSTICS

Regression Analysis by Example by Samprit Chatterjee and Bertram Price (New York: John Wiley & Sons, 1991, 278 pages). A short introductory textbook that provides a very accessible introduction to various issues in multiple regression, including regression diagnostics. All of the essential points are demonstrated by a series of empirical examples.

A First Course in Econometric Theory by Robert Bacon (New York: Oxford University Press, 1989, 336 pages). An econometrics textbook that provides an introduction to regression analysis, including some discussion of estimation procedures for time-series data and structural equation models. The approach is formal but the mathematics are not overly daunting.

Regression: A Second Course in Statistics by Thomas H. Wonnacott and Ronald J. Wonnacott (Malabar, FL: Krieger Publishing Co., 1986, 556 pages). This textbook provides a simple mathematical and graphical introduction to regression analysis, including simple time-series data and structural equation models. It also includes a highly readable discussion of sampling distributions.

Applied Multiple Regression/Correlation Analysis for the Behavioral Sciences by Jacob Cohen and Patricia Cohen (Hillsdale, NJ: Lawrence Erlbaum Associates, 1983, 545 pages). A comprehensive introduction to regression analysis aimed primarily at psychologists. It addresses a variety of practical issues, such as variable transformations, analysis of interaction, and coding schemes for categorical variables.

Regression Diagnostics by John Fox (Newbury Park, CA: Sage Publications, 1991, 92 pages). This handbook provides a concise but accessible introduction to the issue of regression diagnostics, including outliers and influential cases. The discussion employs examples that illustrate the implications of these problems.

TIME-SERIES AND STRUCTURAL EQUATION MODELS

Structural Equations with Latent Variables by Kenneth A. Bollen (New York: John Wiley & Sons, 1989, 514 pages). This textbook provides a comprehensive introduction to a variant of the general linear model that incorporates both observed and unobserved variables. The mathematics may be difficult at points but the empirical examples are easily understood.

Econometric Analysis by William H. Greene (New York: Macmillan Publishing Co., 1990, 783 pages). An advanced econometrics textbook that provides a truly comprehensive introduction to the general linear model, including the analysis of discrete and limited dependent variables. It also includes introductory material on matrix algebra, probability, and sampling distributions.

Time Series Analysis: Regression Techniques by Charles W. Ostrom, Jr. (Newbury Park, CA: Sage Publications, 1990, 94 pages). This short handbook provides a very concise but highly accessible introduction to statistical models for the analysis of time-series data. The discussion relies on empirical examples rather than mathematical derivations.

CATEGORICAL AND LIMITED DEPENDENT VARIABLES

An Introduction to Categorical Data Analysis by Alan Agresti (New York: John Wiley & Sons, 1996, 320 pages). This introductory textbook deals solely with the logic of models for analyzing categorical data. The discussion is geared specifically to those who find the mathematics of these procedures difficult to follow.

Regression Models for Categorical and Limited Dependent Variables by J. Scott Long (Newbury Park, CA: Sage Publications, 1997, 416 pages). A comprehensive introduction to the analysis of categorical and limited dependent variables within the context of the general linear model. It assumes a familiarity with the regression model.

Categorical Data Analysis by Alan Agresti (New York: John Wiley & Sons, 1990, 576 pages). An advanced statistics textbook that discusses the full range of statistical models for analyzing categorical data, especially logit and log-linear models. Although the approach is highly mathematical, most of the discussion is highly accessible.

Index

Printed in the United States
74202LV00003B/129

9 780306 484339